WESTERN PACIFIC EDUCATION IN ACTION SERIES NO. 12

NURSING CARE OF THE SICK

A Guide for Nurses
Working in Small Rural Hospitals

World Health Organization
Regional Office for the Western Pacific
Manila, Philippines
1998

Cataloguing in Publication Data

Nursing care of the sick: A guide for nurses working in small rural hospitals

1.   Nursing care - handbooks.
2.   Patient-centered care.
I.   Hospitals, Rural.

ISBN 92 9061 142 1

The World Health Organization welcomes requests for permission to reproduce or translate its publications, in part or in full. Applications and enquiries should be addressed to the Office of Publications, World Health Organization, Geneva, Switzerland or to the Regional Office for the Western Pacific, Manila, Philippines which will be glad to provide the latest information on any changes made to the text, plans for new editions, and reprints and translations already available.

© World Health Organization 1998

The designations employed and the presentation of the material in this publication do not imply the expression of any opinion whatsoever on the part of the Secretariat of the World Health Organization concerning the legal status of any country, territory, city or area or of its authorities, or concerning the delimitation of its frontiers or boundaries.

The mention of specific companies or of certain manufacturers' products does not imply that they are endorsed or recommended by the World Health Organization in preference to others of a similar nature that are not mentioned.   Errors and omissions excepted, the names of proprietary products are distinguished by initial capital letters.

FOREWORD

Nurses play a vital role in the delivery of health services in every country. Worldwide, at least 50% of all health workers are nurses. In some countries, nurses make up over 80% of the total health workforce.

Nurses play a particularly important role in the delivery of basic health services in rural areas, where they are often the only health workers.

Nurses in these rural communities often provide care under the most difficult circumstances. Many nurses who care for the sick must cope with chronic shortages of essential drugs and basic supplies and equipment. Some rural health facilities lack adequate water supply and sanitary facilities. Most are poorly staffed.

Many of the nursing personnel working in rural areas have had very limited opportunities for training. Most rural health facilities have no books on basic nursing care.

This guide is one of the publications of WHO on its 50th Anniversary. It has been written to support nurses and nursing students working with limited resources in small rural hospitals or health centres. The focus is on the basic care of the sick and injured. The intention is to give practical information which will help nurses to give good nursing care, even where resources are limited.

I hope that this guide will help nurses who are working hard to provide care for the sick in rural communities. We would be pleased to hear from nurses who use this guide and would be grateful for any suggestions about how we can make it more useful in the future.

S.T. Han. MD, Ph.D.
Regional Director

Contents

1

The role of the nurse on the health care team

The patient is the centre of the nurse's concern

Nurses care for the sick and injured in hospitals, where they work to restore health and alleviate suffering. Many people are sent home from the hospital when they still need nursing care, so nurses often provide care in the home that is very similar to the care they give to patients in the hospital. In clinics and health centres in communities which have few doctors, nurses diagnose and treat common illnesses, prescribe and dispense medications and even perform minor surgery. Nurses are also increasingly working to promote people's health and to prevent illness in all communities.

This book focuses on the nurse's roles when people are sick or injured and in the hospital. There are many roles in nursing. The nurse cares for the patient, carries out procedures ordered by the doctor and, in collaboration with the doctor and other team members, assesses the patient and treats his or her problems. The nurse coordinates the work of others involved in caring for the patient, including the patient's family, who may do a lot of the caring for the patient. The nurse also protects the patient, working to prevent infection and ensure a safe, healthy environment in the hospital. Finally, the nurse teaches the patient and family about health-related matters and promotes patients' well-being in all situations, speaking for them (advocating), if necessary. The hospital nurse plays many roles on the health care team.

Care for the patient

Nurses care for patients continuously, 24 hours a day. They help patients to do what they would do for themselves if they could. Nurses take care of their patients, making sure that they can breathe properly, seeing that they get enough fluids and enough nourishment, helping them rest and sleep, making sure that they are comfortable, taking care of their need to eliminate wastes from the body, and helping them to avoid the harmful consequences of being immobile, like stiff joints and pressure sores.

The nurse often makes independent decisions about the care the patient needs based on what the nurse knows about that person and the problems that may occur. For example, the nurse may decide that, in order to prevent pressure sores, the patient needs to be turned every two hours. However, the nurse may consult the doctor about this if it is possible that turning the patient might cause some other problem. Thus the nurse uses understanding of medical conditions, as well as knowledge of nursing, in deciding on patient care.

The nurse not only takes care of the patient but also gives comfort and support to the patient and his or her family. When the patient cannot recover, the nurse helps to make sure that the death is peaceful.

In caring <u>for</u> the patient, the nurse cares <u>about</u> the patient.

> **Caring is the very heart of nursing.**

Work with the doctor to cure the patient

When a person becomes ill or is injured, generally the doctor assesses the patient, diagnoses the patient's problem and decides on the treatment needed to cure the problem or relieve the patient's symptoms. In the past only the doctor assessed and diagnosed. Today, however, nurses play a large role in evaluating patients and detecting problems. In some rural areas, nurses admit patients to hospital and manage their care, referring only the most critical patients to distant medical centres.

In every hospital nurses carry out many of the treatments prescribed for the patient. For example, the doctor may prescribe surgery or bed rest or a certain therapy. The doctor will perform some of these treatments, such as surgery. It is the nurse who gives most of the treatments. If a patient needs intravenous therapy, usually the nurse sets up the intravenous line and gives the patient the fluids and drugs prescribed. If the patient needs an injection, it is the nurse who gives it. The nurse changes the patient's dressings and monitors the healing of the wound. The nurse gives medication for pain. Many physicians order medication for pain "to be given as needed". They let the nurse decide when to give the medication.

The nurse also monitors the patient's progress to make sure that the recovery has no complications. Because nurses have more frequent contact with patients than other staff, they often find problems before anyone else.

 # Coordinate the care of the patient

In taking care of patients, the nurse collaborates with other members of the health care team. The nurse works closely with the doctor, as well as with other nurses, physical therapists, and any other professionals involved in the patient's care. In many hospitals today the team members together plan the care of the patient.

The nurse is the person who coordinates the work of all the team members and sees that the plan is carried out. For example, the nurse makes sure that the patient's appointments for laboratory investigations are made and kept, sees that treatments are given, and checks to be sure that any needed referrals are made before the patient is discharged.

The nurse also plans and supervises the care given by nursing assistants, checks on the work of housekeeping staff assigned to clean the patient's room, and ensures that the patient gets enough healthy food. The family learns how to give basic care from the nurse, who also helps them where necessary. This includes learning how to use traditional ways of healing with modern health care. The nurse supports the family in giving basic care to their sick loved one. It is the nurse who has the final responsibility for the quality of the care the patient receives during the hospital stay.

In coordinating the work of others, the nurse always keeps the patient at the centre of concern.

 ## Protect the patient

When a person is ill and weak, he or she is more vulnerable to infection and injury. One of the major responsibilities of the nurse is to protect the patient by ensuring that the environment is safe and healthy. In particular, the nurse takes every precaution to prevent the spread of infection from one patient to another.

The nurse sees that the patient's room is clean, the patient is clean, water has been boiled or is safe, needles and other materials used for procedures are sterile, soiled materials are kept away from the patient, and needles and other sharp objects are placed in safety containers after use. The nurse washes hands carefully before and after patient care and between patients.

The nurse protects the patient's dignity and tries to save the patient from embarrassment or shame. When the patient's clothing must be removed the nurse tries to ensure the patient's privacy.

4

The nurse also makes sure that the patient is physically safe, cannot fall out of bed, or fall when trying to walk, or slip on a wet floor. The nurse tries to protect the patient against anything that might be harmful in the environment.

> **The nurse protects the patient's privacy.**

 # Teach the patient and family

Teaching is a major role of the nurse in restoring health, promoting health and preventing illness. When a person is ill, the nurse demonstrates things the patient can do to help with recovery. For example, nurses teach patients to cough and breathe deeply after surgery to prevent lung complications. They show patients how to walk on crutches. They teach people with diabetes to monitor their blood sugar.

Whenever the nurse works with a patient, the nurse uses the opportunity to teach that person about self-care. Nurses teach both patients and their families about proper diet and nutrition, cleanliness and hygiene, exercise, sleep and rest and all the other aspects of a healthy life.

Before the patient leaves the hospital, the nurse teaches the patient and family about care at home. For example, nurses teach family members how to bathe the person or wash his or her hair in bed, and how to feed the person or change dressings.

Nurses teach people how to minimize the effects of disability so that they will have the best quality of life.

Advocate for tne patient

Nurses are with people during the most critical times of their lives. Nurses are with people when they are born, when they are injured or ill, when they die. People share the most intimate details of their lives with nurses; they undress for nurses, and trust them to perform painful procedures.

Nurses are at the bedside of the sick and suffering 24 hours a day. They are there when patients cannot sleep because of pain or fear or loneliness. They are there to feed patients, bathe them, and to support them.

Nurses have a long history of caring for the patient and speaking for his or her needs. That is what advocacy is about: supporting the patient, speaking on that person's behalf, and interceding when necessary. This advocacy is a part of the nurse's caring and a part of the closeness and trust between nurse and patient that gives nursing a very special place in health care.

2 Communicating with patients and their families

Communicate with the patient

Illness and hospitalization are stressful, often deeply frightening experiences for patients and their families. The nurse is there to help patients through this experience. Good, clear, supportive communication is an important part of the help given. When you first meet a patient, say, "I am here to help you". Also, immediately tell the patient who you are: "I am Mrs Corpus, your nurse". Then, every time you enter the patient's room, take the opportunity to communicate. Your smile, your caring and your readiness to make contact will ease the patient's time in the hospital. Follow these basic guidelines for communicating with the patient.

Listen to the patient

Begin a conversation with the patient by using open questions like these:

> "How are you feeling today?"

> "Yesterday you were feeling very worried; how are you today?"

Concentrate on the patient and do not let other things distract your attention. Use your eyes, facial expression and tone of voice to show interest. Try not to interrupt. Let the patient say what he or she needs to say.

If the patient's message is not clear, ask questions to get more information or to clarify what was said. Do not jump to conclusions about what the patient means or what the patient needs. Listen to what the patient says and also to how he or she says it and to what is not said. Watch the expressions on the patient's face, and any gestures and body movements. Sometimes the patient's face, or tone of voice, or way of speaking can say more than words.

Keep what the patient says confidential

If information from the patient needs to be given to another person in order to help the patient, let the patient know that you are going to tell that person. For example, if the patient tells you about a symptom that he or she has not had before, tell the patient that you will let the doctor know. If the information will not be useful in helping the patient, do not repeat it to anyone else. Above all, do not gossip about patients with other nurses or other staff.

Put yourself in the patient's place and try to understand what he or she feels

The most important rule in communicating with patients is to imagine yourself in their place. Then you can understand their feelings and respond emotionally to their needs or distress.

The key is to care about the patient as a person, to recognize that this is a human being like you, who is sick and perhaps in pain, who is in need of your help. To express this caring, show warmth and interest when you are with the patient. Be attentive and respectful. Try to meet the patient's needs and respond to his or her feelings.

Remember that when you are kind to another person, both that person's life and yours are enriched.

How to communicate with difficult patients

Sometimes you must deal with patients who are so angry that they shout or angrily criticize you or other nurses or the doctor, refuse the care they need, pull out tubes or pull off bandages. At other times you will encounter patients who complain constantly and want something done for them at every moment. Some patients may scold you or call you incompetent if you do not run to them as soon as they call.

These patients are not easy to like. Often staff respond by becoming angry in return. Sometimes staff simply avoid these patients. Unfortunately, these responses will only make the problems worse.

When patients are angry, it is important to try to find out what they are angry about. Someone may be criticizing the nurse but really be angry that he or she has been diagnosed with a serious disease. It often helps if you calmly ask patients to talk about what their feelings are. It is important to listen and respond with understanding of the pain and difficulties.

If the patient appears to have a legitimate complaint, say that you will tell the nurse or doctor in charge, and do so.

If a patient complains constantly, you can be reassuring in a calm voice, let him or her complain, and perhaps use humour or a smile to help. At the same time, you can set some limits on the patient's demands, while showing warmth and an understanding of the difficulties. For example, you might acknowledge the frustration the person is feeling at having to depend on others for everything.

 # Respond to the patient's needs

Most of the time when patients talk to you, they are conveying information about their feelings and basic needs, and it is important to try to meet those needs as quickly as possible. Patients feel cared about when you try to make them feel better by doing things like bringing water when they ask for it. A smile or a touch that conveys caring and concern for their needs is always helpful.

When the patient gives you information about his or her physical condition, listen carefully and act quickly on the information. If a patient says he or she is in pain, assess the pain and provide relief (see the chapter on caring for the patient in pain). Do not wait an hour to give medication because you have other things to do.

If the patient tells you about new problems, make sure you have the essential information and respond quickly. For example, if the patient says that he or she vomited this morning, try to find out the cause and possible related problems. You might ask such questions as,

> "When did you vomit?
>
> "Did you vomit before or after you ate?"
>
> "Did you feel any nausea before you vomited?"
>
> "Have you felt any nausea before this?"
>
> "Was the vomiting sudden?"
>
> "Have you had any diarrhoea?"

The information in the patient's answers will help you to find out what he or she needs. If the problem appears to be serious, inform the doctor.

Provide information to the patient

When you give information to the patient, be simple and clear. Always be genuine and honest. Do not use medical words to describe the problem or to explain what will be done or what the person can expect to happen. Do not use words that people outside the hospital do not understand. Use ordinary language. Say walk, not ambulate. Do not say you will take an apical pulse. Say you are going to listen to the patient's heart.

Do not pretend that you know things when you do not know. If you cannot answer a patient's question, say that you do not know and offer to try to find the answer. If only the doctor knows the answer, tell the patient that you will ask the doctor, or suggest that the patient ask the doctor.

Never lie to a patient. If the patient is going to feel pain when a tube is removed, do not say that it will not hurt.

The timing of information is important. When the patient is upset, he or she may find it difficult to understand what you are saying. Look and listen carefully before deciding whether the patient is ready to hear you now or if you need to wait.

When you are explaining something to the patient, see if you can tell whether he or she understands what you have said. Ask the person to tell you what he or she heard, or to show you how he or she will do what they have learned. Remember that although patients may smile and nod their head in response, they may be trying to please you. They may not necessarily understand what you said.

Even if you speak very clearly, it is likely that the patient will not understand everything. He or she may forget much of what you say. People who are ill are frightened, and the hospital is a strange and confusing place. Patients who are frightened and confused find it hard to listen carefully. It is easy for them to forget things. You may have to tell the patient more than once.

Some patients want to know a lot about how they are, while others do not. It is important to give patients an opportunity to ask questions and to talk about their fears. If they do not want detailed information, however, do not force it on them.

 # How to give the patient bad news

One of the hardest tasks of doctors and nurses is giving bad news to patients. It is usually the doctor who tells the patient that he or she is not going to recover. Sometimes, however, the patient decides to ask the nurse about it. It is important for the nurse and doctor to talk and agree on how and when to tell the patient. Sometimes the complete truth is too much for the patient. Sometimes it may be best to tell the person a little at a time about what to expect in the future. It is important to know how much the patient understands already and how much he or she wants to understand. Not all patients want to know everything. The best approach is to tell people as much as they indicate they want to know, and then try to help them to deal with their feelings.

When people are told bad news, they often do not want to believe it at first. This is called denial. It is useful as a first response, to help the patient to cope. However, the nurse needs to help the patient move on from denial. The person needs to understand that the situation is real. Gently tell the patient a little at a time about what to expect. Once patients understand what is going to happen, they may become sad and depressed. It is important to recognize their sadness and respond with compassion. It is also important to give patients hope but you must not give them wrong information to make them feel better. To give them hope, you can talk about what may be possible, not about what will definitely happen. You can also give patients hope by telling them that they will have some good time ahead in which they will be able to do many things.

Patients who have difficulty communicating

Sometimes patients cannot communicate clearly. They may not speak the language that is used in the hospital, or they may only speak it a little. You may find that a family member can help, or another staff member may speak the patient's native language. You may work with an interpreter who knows both languages and will translate your questions and the patient's replies. Face the patient and direct your questions to him or her. Carefully watch how the patient looks when speaking. You can understand a lot about what the patient means or is feeling even without words. Do not ignore the interpreter. Let the interpreter translate the questions while you face the patient.

Sometimes patients are deaf, blind or have poor vision. If patients cannot hear well, watch if they are reading your lips or if they are trying to communicate with sign language. If they are using their hands to communicate and you do not understand, try to find a family member to help you.

Sometimes a patient is confused, or cannot form words, or find the right words. When a person has a tube inserted he or she cannot speak at all. With these patients, try to communicate without using words. Ask the patient to signal yes or no to questions by using hand squeezes, or head movements, or eye blinks. Or give the patient paper or a word board to write on.

If the patient is trying to communicate but you do not understand, say that you do not understand, but provide support and encouragement, and continue the conversation. Do not pretend to understand when you do not. When the patient cannot communicate with you in words, it is especially important that you show attentiveness, warmth and respect through your touch and smiles.

How to communicate with families

Families of patients have to make many adjustments and changes in response to the illness, particularly if it is very serious and lasting. For example, they may have to spend time doing the tasks the sick person did before in the family. They also spend time going to visit and trying to take care of the sick person both in the hospital and when he or she returns home. They may lose money because of this sickness. The family members may be under a lot of stress. This may make them angry and difficult at times. When this happens it is important to think about how they are feeling. Try to realize how hard the situation is for them.

Make time to talk to the patient's family as soon as the patient is admitted; the sooner the better. Answer their questions simply but clearly. If they want more information than you can give them, offer to call the doctor or help to find a time when they can talk to the doctor. Ask the family about the patient; family members have a lot of useful information.

Whenever the family comes to visit, tell them what has been happening to their family member. Offer support and encouragement. Do not lie to the family. If they want to know more than you feel free to tell them, try to help them to talk with the doctor.

If the news is bad, you may wish to tell the family first and ask them to take part in a discussion about the best way to tell the patient. You may decide with the doctor that the patient should be told first, and then the family. Sometimes families want to help decide what will be done with their family member. For example, they want to help decide whether he or she will have surgery for the cancer. When they know what is expected to happen they might feel that it is better to do nothing at all except care for the person's symptoms.

If a family member wants to stay with the patient, make this as easy as possible.

If the family wish to help to care for the patient, give them instructions on providing daily care.

Before the patient leaves the hospital, talk to the family about the care he or she will need at home. Make sure they are able to give it. (This is discussed further in the chapter on preparing the patient for discharge.)

3

Monitoring the patient and recording nursing care

Nurses see the patient more than any other care provider. Therefore, nurses are in the best position to monitor the patient's progress, spot problems early and judge what care is needed to solve the problem. To do these things the nurse must use every opportunity to assess the patient, always asking the question, "What is happening to this patient?".

> **Whenever you enter the patient's room, carefully look at how the patient is, check all the equipment in the room, and check the environment of the room.**

Here are some basic guidelines to use when you are checking what is happening to the patient.

Get background information

Before you go into a patient's room, check the chart to see what has been done today, what problems other caregivers have noted, and whether there is any other new information available about the patient. If possible, talk about this with the nurse who is going off duty.

Observe the patient

- Listen to the patient's breathing, look at his or her colour, and see whether the patient is awake.

- Immediately take the patient's vital signs if you see any signs that the patient is having trouble breathing, is breathing too fast, or his or her colour is unnaturally pale or reddish, or if the patient appears to be in distress. Report problems to the nurse in charge or the doctor.

- Do not wake up the patient for assessment or care unless the breathing or colour indicates a problem. If the patient's breathing, colour, or position in the bed suggests unconsciousness rather than normal sleep, try to wake up the patient. If you cannot rouse him or her, call for help. At the same time, make sure that the patient's airway is open; if necessary, open it by lifting the lower jaw.

 # Talk with the patient

- If the patient is awake, ask how he or she is and whether he or she is comfortable.

- Ask about any pain.

- Ask whether the treatment or medication given has helped.

- Ask whether the patient has been eating and drinking.

- Ask about urinary and faecal elimination.

- Note any problems the patient mentions.

If the person does not volunteer information, ask specifically about symptoms that you might expect to find, such as fatigue, nausea, or respiratory problems. If family members are present, it is helpful also to ask them how the patient seems and whether they have noted any problems. Ask them also about what the patient has eaten and drunk.

Examine the patient

Examine the patient briefly from head to toe, noting any changes or abnormalities. Pay particular attention to the problems which brought the patient into the hospital.

What you look for will depend on what the problem is and what body systems are affected by it.

 # Check any equipment in use

The checks you make will depend on what the patient's problem is and what equipment is being used for the problem; it may be an oxygen system, a nasogastric tube, an indwelling catheter, or an intravenous line, for example.

If the patient is receiving oxygen:

Make sure that the cannula or catheter is properly placed.

Check that the oxygen is humidified and running at the ordered number of litres per minute. Check also that there is enough oxygen in the tank.

If the patient has an intravenous line:

Make sure the intravenous line is open and the correct solution is flowing at the correct rate.

Check the site where the catheter enters the skin for any redness, warmth, or signs that the solution may be leaking from the vein out into the tissues. If the skin is swollen or pale at the site and the patient feels pain, it is likely that the fluid has gone into the tissues and the intravenous line must be taken out and put in again.

If the patient has a foley catheter in place:

Check the urine output. Look at whether the urine is clear, cloudy, reddish, or dark and concentrated.

Check the intake and output record to help you to work out the patient's fluid status.

Make sure that the foley catheter tubing is not twisted. The foley bag should not be resting on the floor.

 ## Assess the patient's environment

It is the nurse's responsibility to see that the patient's environment is clean and safe.

- Check the overall cleanliness of the room and floor. Make sure the floor is dry.

- Check the patient's bed and the area around it. Make sure that the bedding is clean and smooth and the area around the bed is clean and tidy. Dirty eating equipment and soiled tissue can be a source of infection for the patient and the nurse.

- Check that the toilet area is clean. If possible, see that the patient has soap and a towel for washing.

- Check that the patient has what he or she needs.

- If the patient is able to drink fluids, make sure that there is fresh water by the bed.

Take the patient's vital signs

> ## Vital signs are vital.

One of the most important aspects of assessing the patient is taking the vital signs. The patient's vital signs are temperature, pulse, breathing (respiration) and blood pressure. Changes in any of the vital signs can indicate changes in the patient's condition. Large or sudden changes should always be reported to the doctor.

- Vital signs should be checked on admission and at regular intervals after that. In many hospitals they are checked every four hours.

- When patients are in intensive care or have just come back from surgery, their vital signs are checked more frequently.

- Vital signs should also be checked:

  - before and after any invasive procedure

  - before and after giving any medication that can affect blood pressure or respiration

  - before and after any nursing procedure that might affect any vital signs, for example, walking a patient who has been on bed rest.

Always check vital signs when a patient complains of light-headedness, dizziness, being suddenly hot, or whenever the patient's condition changes for the worse.

Temperature

The body temperature is the heat of the body measured in degrees. The average temperature of an adult measured orally is between 36.7°C and 37°C.

A temperature higher than the usual average is called a fever or hyperthermia. At its first appearance, the signs of fever include:

- an increased pulse
- increased breathing
- shivering
- cold skin
- feelings of being cold (having a chill).

Clinical alert: Extremely high fevers can cause convulsions. They can damage the liver, kidneys and other organs and even cause death.

During the course of the fever, clinical signs include:

- skin that feels warm to the touch
- continued increased pulse rate and breathing
- thirst
- dehydration
- loss of appetite
- a general feeling of unease
- drowsiness, restlessness and, in severe cases, delirium.

When a fever begins to go down, the patient still feels warm and is flushed and sweating; the person may also be dehydrated but does not have chills.

A body temperature which is lower than the average is called hypothermia. The clinical signs include:

- severe shivering
- pale, cool, waxy skin
- low blood pressure (hypotension)
- decreased urinary output

- disorientation
- in severe cases, drowsiness and coma.

The nurse routinely takes the patient's temperature to check for infection. **Fever is a sign of infection**. If a patient has a fever, the nurse checks the temperature to see whether fever is continuing, getting worse, or whether the medication has reduced the temperature. The nurse also takes the temperature to see whether the care given has changed it.

The body temperature can be measured at oral, rectal and axillary (under the arm) sites. It can also be measured in the ear at the tympanic membrane (ear drum).

A mercury thermometer is generally used to measure temperature. The thermometer may have a long slender tip or a rounded tip. The slender tip is best for oral or axillary temperature; the rounded tip is used to take rectal temperature.

To read a mercury thermometer, hold it at eye level and turn it until you can see the mercury line. The upper end of the line, the highest point the mercury has reached, gives the temperature.

How to take an oral temperature

A person's temperature is usually measured in the mouth, or orally. This is the easiest way to take a temperature. If the patient is under five years old or is confused, the temperature must be taken another way in case he or she bites the thermometer and breaks it. If a patient has had cold or hot fluids or has been smoking, you must wait 15 to 30 minutes before taking an oral temperature to make sure that the temperature reading is accurate.

- Wash your hands.
- Shake the thermometer down to below 35°C.
- Put the thermometer under the patient's tongue, to the right or left of the pocket at the base of the tongue.

- Tell the patient to close his or her lips, but not the teeth, around the thermometer. Leave the thermometer in place for at least three minutes.

- Take out the thermometer and read the temperature.

- Wash the thermometer in soapy lukewarm water (never hot), rinse it in cold water, wipe it with disinfectant and store it dry.

- Wash your hands and record the temperature.

How to take an axillary temperature

To take an axillary temperature, the thermometer is put under the patient's arm (in the axilla). This is not the most accurate way to take a temperature, but it is done for adults who have inflammation of the mouth and patients who are confused. An axillary temperature is usually a half degree lower than an oral temperature.

- Wash your hands.

- Prepare the thermometer just as you would to take an oral temperature.

- Put the thermometer under the patient's arm in the axilla.

- Ask the patient to hold the arm tight against the chest and leave the thermometer in place for five minutes in children and nine minutes in adults.

- Take out the thermometer, read the temperature and clean and store the thermometer.

- Wash your hands and record the temperature.

How to take a rectal temperature

Rectal temperatures are considered the most accurate. They are usually taken only with infants and children who cannot yet hold a thermometer in their mouth without breaking it. A rectal temperature is usually a degree higher than an oral temperature.

When you take a rectal temperature, use a thermometer with a rounded tip.

- Wash your hands.

- Ask the patient to lie on his or her side, with knees flexed. A child should lie on one side or prone, on your lap.

- Check the temperature recorded on the thermometer. If it reads more than 35°C, shake it down.

- Put some lubricant on a tissue and then onto the first 2.5 cm of the thermometer. The lubricant makes it easier not to irritate the membranes when you put in the thermometer.

- Ask the patient to take a deep breath and put the thermometer into the anus from 1.5 to 4 cm depending on the patient's age and size. Do not force the thermometer.

- Hold the thermometer in place for two minutes.

- Remove the thermometer, wipe it with a tissue, and discard the tissue. Read the thermometer.

- Wash and rinse the thermometer, wipe it with disinfectant, dry it and store it dry.

- Wash your hands.

- Record the temperature.

How to take the patient's pulse

The heart is a pump that pushes blood into the arteries. With each heartbeat, there is a pulsing pressure as the blood goes into the arteries. The pulse therefore reflects the heartbeat. A normal adult pulse usually is from 60 to 80 beats a minute, but the range is 60 to 100.

The pulse is faster in women than in men. It is much faster in children than in adults. The pulse increases with exercise and with stress, and when the patient has a fever. The pulse is also faster when the patient is losing blood. Some medications decrease the pulse rate and others increase it.

It is important to take the patient's pulse to find out whether it is in the normal range, and whether it is regular or not. Most of the time the pulse is taken on the thumb side of the inner wrist; this is called the radial pulse.

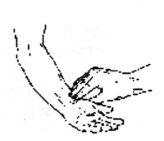

The radial pulse is on the thumb side of the wrist

A pulse can also be taken at several other places on the body. If you cannot get to the radial pulse because the patient has a bandage there, or you need to assess the pulse in a particular part of the body, use another site. Any pulse taken away from the heart is called a peripheral pulse.

To take the patient's peripheral pulse, whether on the wrist or at another site, you need a clock or a watch with a second hand.

- Use your index and middle fingertips or all three middle fingertips and apply moderate pressure over the pulse point, until you feel the pulsing. Never use your thumb because you have a pulse in your thumb that you could mistake for the patient's pulse.

- Count the number of beats for a full minute. After that, if the pulse is normal, count for 30 seconds and multiply by two.

- Note whether the pulse is weak, normal, or too strong (bounding).

- Note whether the pulse is regular or not.

- If the pulse is faster or slower than usual for this patient, or the pulse is irregular or bounding or weak, report this to the nurse or doctor in charge.

How to take an apical pulse

Sometimes a pulse may be so weak that you cannot hear it unless you listen to it near the heart. A pulse taken at the apex of the heart is called the apical pulse.

To take an apical pulse, you need a stethoscope and a watch which shows the seconds.

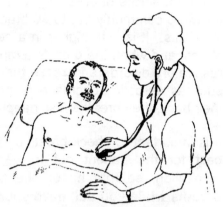

Taking an apical pulse

- Wash your hands.

- Use an antiseptic wipe to clean the earpieces and diaphragm (the flat-edged piece of the stethoscope) if they are soiled.

- Find the pulse site on the left side of the chest.

- Put the earpieces of the stethoscope in your ears, with the ear pieces pointing or facing forward.

- Put the diaphragm over the apical pulse and listen for heart sounds, which sound like "lub dub "

- Note whether the spaces between heart sounds are regular or not. This is the rhythm of the heart beat.

- Note the strength or weakness (volume) of the heartbeat.

- Count the heartbeats for 30 seconds and multiply by 2 if the rhythm is regular; count them for 60 seconds if the pulse is irregular. This is the pulse rate.

- Wash your hands.

- Record the pulse rate, rhythm and strength.

Check the patient's breathing

The normal rate of breathing, or respiration, in a resting adult is 12 (or more commonly 15) to 20 breaths a minute. The rate is higher in infants. It is also higher in a person who is exercising or under stress, and when the outside temperature is higher. Infections and respiratory disorders increase the rate as well. Some medications such as narcotics decrease respiration. When people lie flat on their back, they breathe less deeply.

It is important to check breathing when the patient is resting. It is best for the patient not to be aware that you are checking respiration, so that he or she breathes as usual. **Count the breaths while you still have your fingers on the patient's pulse, as if you were continuing to count the pulse. The patient will not notice that you are actually checking the breathing.**

- To check the **rate** of breathing, count the number of breaths for at least a minute.

- To check the **rhythm**, note whether the spaces between breaths are regular or not.

- To check the **depth** of breathing, look at the movement of the person's chest or place your hand on the person's chest to feel the movement. When the person breathes in, the ribs move upward and outward so that the lungs can expand; when the person breathes out, the ribs move in as the lungs are compressed. If there is a lot of movement of the chest, the breathing is deep; if the movement is very little, the breathing is shallow.

- Look at the amount of **effort** the patient has to make in order to breathe, and listen to the sound of the person's breathing. Normal breathing is silent and easy. Sometimes the patient is clearly working to breathe, particularly when he or she is lying flat. If the patient is working hard, you will often see tightness of the neck and shoulder muscles. Sometimes you will see that the skin has been pulled in above the sternum or below the ribs (called insuction or retraction).

- Listen for wheezing, which is a whistling or sighing sound. Wheezing is a sign of serious infection, asthma, or a blockage in the airway.

- Write down what you notice about the patient's breathing. If you see any changes in the patient, tell the nurse in charge or the doctor immediately.

> *Clinical alert.*
> **Always report fast breathing. It is a sign that something is wrong. It can mean that the patient has an infection such as pneumonia, heart failure, blood loss or other problems.**

How to take blood pressure

Blood pressure is a measure of the pressure that the blood makes as it moves through the body's arteries. There are two kinds of blood pressure: systolic pressure and diastolic pressure.

- Systolic pressure is the highest pressure produced when the left ventricle of the heart contracts. It is the pressure of the wave of blood going into the arteries.

- Diastolic pressure is the lowest pressure produced when the left ventricle relaxes. It is the pressure that is always within the arteries.

- Blood pressure is measured in millimetres of mercury (mm Hg) and is usually given as the systolic pressure followed by the diastolic pressure, with a slash between.

Example of blood pressure:

systolic → **140** diastolic
pressure 90 ← pressure

- The normal blood pressure of an adult ranges from 110/60 to 140/90 mm Hg, and the average is 120/80 mm Hg.

High blood pressure or hypertension is pressure that continues to be above 140/90 mm Hg.

Low blood pressure or hypotension is systolic pressure that is below 100 mm Hg.

It is important to know the patient's normal blood pressure in order to see changes that may show problems.

Blood pressure is measured with a blood pressure cuff, a sphygmomanometer, and a stethoscope.

The stethoscope is used to listen to the sounds of the blood in the artery.

Take the blood pressure in the patient's arm using the brachial artery, which is the artery in the middle of the elbow crease.

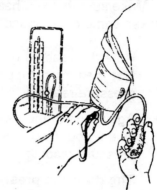

Place stethoscope over the brachial pulse in the elbow crease

- To begin, wash your hands.

- Put the patient in a comfortable position, sitting or lying on one side, with the arm to be measured slightly bent and supported. The cuff should be at the level of the heart.

- Wrap the cuff around the upper arm and fasten it. The bladder inside the cuff has to be directly over the artery. The lower border of the cuff should be about 2.5 cm above the elbow crease (called the antecubital space).

- Feel the artery with your fingertips. It should be in the centre of the antecubital space. This is called the brachial pulse.

- While you are feeling the brachial pulse with one hand, close the valve and pump up the cuff with the other hand. Pump until the reading on the sphygmomanometer is 30 mm above the point where the brachial pulse disappears.

- Put the diaphragm of the stethoscope over the brachial artery.

- Release the valve on the cuff slowly so that the pressure goes down at the rate of 2-3 mm per second.

- Listen for the sounds.

The systolic pressure is the pressure at which you first hear tapping sounds. Make sure that you hear two sounds, to be sure you have not mistaken some other sound for the blood sound.

- Note the reading on the sphygmomanometer when you first hear the tapping sounds. That is the systolic pressure reading.

- Again, note the reading on the sphygmomanometer when you hear the last sound; that is the diastolic pressure reading.

  The diastolic pressure is the point at which the very last sound is heard.

- Release the valve and deflate the cuff quickly.

- Remove the cuff from the patient's arm and record the blood pressure readings, with the systolic first and the diastolic second.

- If there are any significant changes in blood pressure from the last time it was measured, report this immediately.

Plan the nursing care

After checking how the patient is (the status), plan the care you will give this day.

The plan of care will include:

- procedures ordered by the doctor
- nursing measures to provide comfort and promote recovery.

Record the patient's status and nursing care

Recording or noting information is an essential part of nursing care. After you have checked the patient and provided care, you need to note three types of information:

- important information about the status of the patient

- the care you gave the patient

- the patient's response to your care.

The main reason for writing down information about the patient is so that the caregiver who follows you knows what has been happening. The next caregiver needs to know how the patient was before, to see if anything has changed. For example, you take vital signs not only to decide whether the patient has a problem needing your immediate attention, but also to provide baseline data for the nurse who follows you. Then when that nurse takes vital signs, he or she can quickly see whether they are stable or whether there are changes that need to be watched or which need to be dealt with immediately.

Write a nurse's note only about what you think is important. A nurse's note might look like this:

Date	Time	
15/9/97	0800	Dressing changed and drainage checked. Wound is clean. Patient says she is in less pain than yesterday but continues to be nauseated. S. Ramos, RN

It is very important to write your notes as soon as you leave the patient. If you wait until later, you will forget what you have seen or done or you will confuse what you saw in this patient with what you saw in others. Never wait to record.

Evaluate the care given

After caring for the patient, always go back to see if your nursing care has been effective. For example, if you give the patient medication for pain, go back to see if the patient is feeling more comfortable.

If your nursing measures have not been effective, you may need to plan and carry out other measures to help the patient.

Reminder

The patient's status should be assessed every time the nurse gives care.

Your observations and the information you gather from the patient help you to decide whether the patient is getting better or is experiencing problems that need attention.

4 Daily care of the patient

The basic activities of daily life are eating, dressing, bathing, going to the toilet, sleeping and resting, walking and communicating with others. Often when people are sick, they cannot do all these things alone and they need your help. When people are very ill, you may have to do nearly everything for them. In many hospitals, the family may give most of this care, with the guidance and supervision of the nurse.

This chapter describes some of the procedures the nurse or family members use to help patients with the activities of daily living and to assure their comfort.

Helping the patient to walk and get exercise is described in the chapter on caring for the patient with limited mobility. Helping the patient to eat well is in the chapter on meeting patients' nutritional needs. Helping the patient with elimination (going to the toilet) is in the chapter on caring for the patient who has problems with elimination. Communication is covered in the chapter on communicating with patients and their families.

Hygiene

It is important to help the patient to stay clean and to take care of the skin, mouth, hair, eyes, ears, and nails. When a person is ill, it is hard to think about bathing or brushing the teeth or cleaning the nails; breathing or coping with pain seem a lot more important. Therefore, the nurse needs to look at whether the patients can clean themselves and help them when necessary. It is important to ask patients what they usually do and how they prefer to be helped.

Different cultures and different religions may have different hygiene practices. Hygiene is very personal and individuals have different ideas about what they want to do. When possible, the nurse should help patients to meet their own personal needs rather than carrying out a standard routine.

Bathing

Healthy skin is important. It protects the tissues from injury by preventing germs (microorganisms) from entering the body. When the skin is scratched or broken, microorganisms can enter and the patient is vulnerable to infection. When the skin is dry or flaky, it may crack. When the patient has a rash or other itching, it is easy to scratch the skin.

It is therefore important always to check the patient's skin. Avoid injuring the skin and improve skin health if possible, through nutrition, lotions and above all, bathing.

Bathing removes microorganisms from the skin as well as body secretions, gets rid of unpleasant smells, improves blood circulation to the skin and makes the patient feel more relaxed and refreshed.

Patients may be bathed every day in the hospital. However, if a patient's skin is dry, bathing may be limited to once or twice a week so that it does not dry out further.

The nurse or a family member may need to help the patient walk to the shower or tub and to go back. Have a chair ready at the shower, in case the patient needs to sit and rest. The nurse or family member should be available to help the patient wash or dry off, if needed, or change into clean clothes after bathing.

Sometimes patients can wash themselves in bed. Sometimes they need some help from the nurse or a family member, for example, in washing their back or feet. Sometimes patients cannot wash themselves and the nurse or family member washes them in bed.

Bathing the patient gives the nurse a good opportunity to look at the condition of the patient's skin and to see how well the patient can move.

Before beginning a bed bath, try to avoid draughts by closing windows or doors, if necessary, and do all you can to give the patient privacy.

Have ready a basin of warm water, soap, a cloth for washing and one for rinsing, a bath blanket or sheet and two towels, if available, one to dry the patient with and the other to cover part of the body as you wash. You should change the bath water at least once and preferably twice if enough water is available.

Mouth care

Good mouth care requires daily tooth brushing, massage of the gums and rinsing out the mouth. Patients in hospital may be able to get up and brush their teeth and wash out their mouth. If the nurse brings a toothbrush and basin of water, patients can sit up in bed and brush their teeth there. However, sometimes a patient is too ill to take care of his or her mouth; as a result, it can become dry or irritated or develop a bad smell. These problems may be increased by the illness or by the medicines the patient is taking.

The nurse needs to check the patient's mouth every day and either help the person to care for it or do the mouth care for him or her. Usually mouth care should be done daily. Depending on the condition of the patient's mouth, this care may be needed more often.

It is particularly important to do frequent mouth care for a patient who is receiving nothing by mouth.

As you do mouth care, always look for bleeding or ulcerations and ask the patient about any pain.

The type of mouth care the nurse gives will depend on the supplies available. When possible, the teeth and gums should be gently brushed with a soft toothbrush. If a toothbrush is not available, the patient can chew on the fibres at the end of a stick, using them as a brush, or you can wrap a piece of rough towel around the end of a stick or your finger and use it as a toothbrush. Toothpaste is helpful but not necessary.

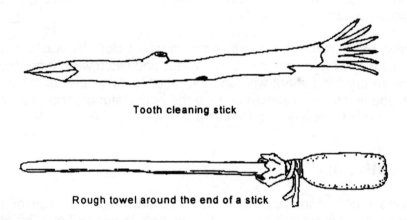

Tooth cleaning stick

Rough towel around the end of a stick

You can make a tooth powder by mixing salt and bicarbonate of soda (or ashes) in equal amounts. To make it stick, wet the brush before putting it in the powder.

If patients have false teeth (dentures) and they are unable to clean them, ask them to take the teeth out each night. Brush them with a toothbrush and toothpaste or a tooth powder you have made, rinse them, and put them in a container by the patient's bed.

Even helping people to rinse out their mouth with salt solution or clean water will help to prevent dryness and infection and make them feel more comfortable.

If the mouth membranes look dry or dirty, put some oil and lemon juice, if available, on a gauze pad or clean cloth, and wipe the membranes. A little oil on the lips will help to prevent dryness and painful cracking.

Mouth care for the unconscious patient

Mouth care is especially important for an unconscious patient. Special precautions need to be taken.

- If possible, position the patient on his or her side, near the edge of the bed.

- Wash your hands.

- Put a little basin under the patient's chin with a towel under it to catch any water that drips.

- Open the patient's mouth very gently with a tongue blade or other object, such as a spoon.

- Clean the teeth and membranes, then rinse the mouth by injecting a little water into the mouth with a syringe. Or use a moistened swab or cloth to rinse the mouth.

- If you inject water into the patient's mouth, make sure that it all runs out of the side of the mouth or suction the mouth to get it out. Fluid left in the mouth could choke the patient. It could be breathed into the lungs and cause pneumonia.

- After cleaning the patient's mouth, wash your hands.

 # Hair care

Hair needs brushing or combing every day to stay healthy. Many patients are able to get up and comb their hair, or comb it in bed. If the patient cannot comb or brush his or her own hair, the nurse or a family member needs to do it, at least once daily.

Hair washing generally depends on its oiliness and the person's preferences. A patient in hospital for a long time will need to have a hair wash. Patients who can bathe themselves can also shampoo their hair. Other patients may be able to sit up in a chair in front of the sink. The nurse or a relative can then shampoo their hair.

Some patients are not able to get up to bathe or wash their hair and the nurse will need to shampoo it in bed. Ask the patient to move close to the side of the bed, and bring shampoo and two basins of water. Put a towel under the patient's head and shoulders to keep the bed dry. Wet the hair, put on the shampoo and wash the hair, massaging the scalp with your fingertips. Then rinse the hair, dry it with a clean towel, and comb it out to prevent tangles.

 ## Shaving the male patient

Usually male patients who are too ill to shave their faces will feel much more comfortable if you or a family member gives a shave when needed.

- To prevent infection, it is best not to share razors between patients. If the patient's family can provide a razor, ask them to bring one.

- Wash your hands before beginning the shave.

- Moisten the patient's face with a warm wet washcloth. Then put soap or shaving lotion on one side of his face at a time.

- Shave gently, following the direction of the hair.

- While shaving the patient, be careful of the skin creases near the mouth and nose. These areas are best shaved in short strokes while carefully stretching the skin flat with your left hand.

- When you have finished, rinse the patient's face with warm water.

- Wash your hands.

Eye care

Usually a person's eyes do not require any special care since they are continually cleaned by the fluid in the eyes, and the eyelashes and eyelids stop particles from getting into the eyes. However, a patient who has had an eye injury or surgery, a patient who has an eye infection, or an unconscious patient may need special care of the eyes. With infections or injuries, the eyes tend to drain and the discharge may accumulate and dry on the lashes like a crust. Unconscious patients may not blink and their eyes may become dry and irritated. Discharge from the eyes may also build up.

When you care for the patient, check the condition of the eyes and lashes.

- Soften and wipe away any discharge that has dried on the eyelids or lashes, using a sterile cotton ball or clean cloth moistened with water or saline solution. Wipe from the inner part of the eyelid to the outer part.

- If the patient is unconscious and cannot close the eyelids or blink, eye drops can be used to keep the eye wet enough. Or put an eye patch over the eye to protect it.

- If the patient wears glasses, clean them carefully with warm water and a soft tissue or cloth to avoid scratching the lens. When they are not being used, they should be kept in a place where they will not get broken.

Care of the ears

Normally, ears need very little cleaning. However, a patient with too much earwax may need his or her ears cleaned so the doctor or nurse can see inside the ear.

When you are caring for the patient, check the patient's ears for drainage, build-up of earwax, or inflammation. Wipe out the ears with a clean wash cloth and remove the excess wax. Usually you can loosen the wax by pulling the ear lobe downward. If the wax can still not be dislodged, you may need to irrigate the ear canal.

Clinical alert: **Never irrigate a patient's ear if the ear drum is perforated.**

You will need an irrigating solution at room temperature, a container for the solution, a syringe or a bulb suction, a small basin to catch the liquid, a towel, and cotton balls, if available.

- Wash your hands.
- Fill the syringe or bulb suction with the irrigating solution, and gently pull the ear lobe up and back to straighten out the ear canal, so that the solution can flow through the whole canal.
- Insert the tip of the syringe or bulb suction into the ear and very gently direct the solution into the canal. Let the solution drip out and be sure the syringe does not block it.
- When you have finished, wipe the outside of the ear and ask the patient to turn onto one side with the ear down, so that the rest of the solution will drain out. Put a towel under the ear to keep the bed dry.

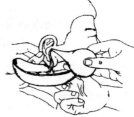

Irrigating the ear

 # Nail care

Some patients may need help in cleaning or cutting fingernails and toe nails. Using a nail cutter or sharp scissors, cut the fingernail straight across and then use a nail file, if available, to round off the nail. When you have cut all the nails, gently clean under them. If the patient has diabetes or problems with circulation, or an infected finger, you must be very careful not to injure the tissues.

If the patient's toenails are thick and hard, you may need to soak the foot in a basin before cutting the nails. Check both fingernails and toenails for any signs of inflammation.

 # Care of the legs and feet

Always check the patient's lower legs and feet, especially if the patient is elderly or has diabetes or circulatory problems. The patient may have poor sensation and circulation but may not know that. The patient then may not know about sores or ulcers on his or her feet or toes.

Look at and feel the lower legs and feet. If the skin of the lower legs is brownish and thick, or if it is red and shiny, the patient may have circulatory problems. Check the presence and strength of pulses in the feet (pedal pulses). Check the colour and temperature of the feet and toes. Check for swelling of the feet, ankles, and lower legs. Look between the toes and at the bottoms of the feet.

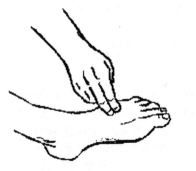 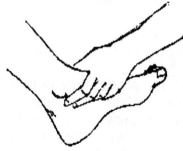

Dorsalis pedis   *Posterior tibialis pulse*

Clinical alert:

Danger signs showing circulatory loss, severe infection or gangrene must be reported immediately to the doctor. These signs are:

- ulcer or infected area with a bad smell
- area painful to touch
- a cool or cold, bluish limb or foot
- white or hard black skin or skin coming off
- decreased or absent pulses
- warm, red streaks from an ulcer or infection running upward
- the patient looks very ill.

If there is a sore or ulcer, get an order for treatment. Calluses can be softened by soaking the feet in warm water, then shaving the callus. If the patient has dry skin, bathe the feet or moisten them with warm water. Dry well between the toes. Apply oil or lotion, rubbing it in well. Do not apply lotion between the toes.

Giving a foot massage after bathing or caring for the feet can be very relaxing for the patient.

Tell the patient how to care for any deformities, sores, ulcers or poor circulation or sensation in the feet and legs. The patient or a family member should examine the feet every day and keep them clean and dry. When the patient goes home, he or she should not go barefoot. If there are any burns, blisters or sores, the patient should be seen by a health care worker.

Back rubs

A back rub is one of the most comforting things you can do for patients. It relieves tension, relaxes the patient and improves circulation. Because of its effects on circulation, the back rub is particularly useful in preventing pressure sores in those on bed rest. It also allows the nurse to check the patient's skin and look for red areas that may later develop pressure sores. But massage should be used cautiously. If skin is reddened, massage may cause more damage.

The best times to give a back rub are after a bath or before the patient goes to sleep.

A lotion may be used to soften the skin during the massage. Alcohol is refreshing, but it is not usually recommended because it dries out the skin. First wash your hands. Then pour a little lotion into your hands and warm it by holding it for a few seconds before beginning the rub. Now, using circular motions, massage the middle of

> *Clinical alert:* **Do not rub over reddened areas of the skin since rubbing skin can cause pressure sores to form.**

the patient's lower back. Next stroke upward and massage the areas over the right and left shoulder blades, again using circular motions. Then stroke downward and end by massaging the iliac crests, the large muscles of the right and left buttocks. Repeat this process for three to five minutes, and then take off any lotion left on the skin with a towel.

When you are massaging the back, check the skin for redness that does not go away after being rubbed. These are areas to watch, since they may develop into pressure sores.

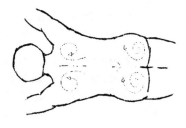

Back rub

How to prevent and treat pressure sores

Pressure sores or decubitus ulcers are among the complications of bed rest. They usually form on bony parts of the body such as the elbows and hips, knees, and the sacrum or big bone at the back of the pelvis. The area first looks red, then an open sore develops.

If the ulcer is not treated, the damage continues and the tissues below the skin are affected, then even the muscle and bone are involved. Untreated sores may easily become infected.

A mobile patient is less likely to develop pressure sores. It is important to move and turn the patient, exercise his or her joints, and get the patient up and walking as soon as possible.

Ways to avoid pressure sores:

- **Help the patient change position every one to two hours.**

- **Keep the patient well nourished.** See that he or she gets enough calories, protein and vitamin C.

- **Keep the patient clean.** If the skin is not clean, bacteria will collect and make pressure sores develop more quickly.

- **Keep the patient dry.** Moisture from urine and perspiration helps pressure sores to form.

- **Keep bedding clean and free of wrinkles.** This will reduce friction, which also leads to pressure sores.

- **If necessary, use a foam rubber pad or soft mattress.** This will reduce the pressure on bony parts of the body such as the back of the pelvis (sacrum). Raising the heels makes them less likely to develop sores.

Every time you give care to a patient who is on bed rest or has limited mobility, check bony parts of the body for the signs of pressure sores, so that you can begin treatment. Early signs include red or pale skin or local swelling and a tingling or burning sensation. Encourage the patient to change position as often as possible if any of these signs are present, and exercise the area to stimulate blood circulation.

How to treat pressure sores:

- Once a sore develops, it should be carefully cleaned and dressed. Use the aseptic technique described in the chapter on protecting the patient from infection. The sore can be washed with saline solution or hydrogen peroxide, and an ointment applied. If it is not infected, it should then be covered with a dressing that stops air reaching the sore and keeps in body moisture. Leave the dressing in place for several days without disturbing it to prevent infection and promote healing. If the sore is already infected, put on an antibiotic ointment or solution. If the sore has a scab or dry crust on it, it may have to be softened with saline solution before it can be removed. Once it is soft, remove it with scissors and forceps. Clean the sore with saline solution and apply ointment.

- Reposition the patient at least every two hours to keep pressure off the sore spot, and encourage the patient to shift his or her weight, if only slightly, as often as possible.

- If the sore has developed on the patient's pelvis, keep the bed flat or the head raised no more than 30 degrees, to prevent friction and added pressure to the pelvic area.

Help the patient get enough rest and sleep

When people are sick, they often need more rest and sleep than they would normally because the body is spending a great deal of energy on healing. Unfortunately, many aspects of illness also make it harder to get rest and sleep. People who have shortness of breath or congestion often find it hard to sleep. Patients with pain are often woken up by it. A patient who is anxious will also have more trouble sleeping. Being in a strange place such as the hospital makes it harder to sleep. Hospitals tend to be noisy at times when the patient is used to quiet.

To prepare patients for sleep, make sure they have enough blankets to be warm and their clothes are comfortable. Help them to go to the toilet before bedtime, so that they are not woken up in the night. Give pain medication 30 minutes before bed time so that pain will not keep them awake. Unless the patient has such severe pain that he or she must get medication during the night to control it, try to avoid giving any more medications until morning. It is always helpful to offer patients a back rub just before they go to sleep.

Staff and relatives should keep the patient's area as quiet as possible. Staff conversations nearby should be kept to a minimum. Hall lights should be dimmed or turned off. Conversations at the nurse's station should be carried on quietly. Avoid loud conversations or loud noises. Make sure that all radios are turned off during sleeping hours.

 # Ensure the patient's safety

Patients in the hospital can easily fall because they are weak and their protective senses may not be as good as usual. To prevent falls, the floors in the patient's room, the toilet and the halls must be kept clean and dry. A patient may easily slip on a wet floor. Also, keep the patient's area and the toilet clear. The patient needs an open walkway.

Some patients may need restraints to stop them from falling out of bed. Side rails on the beds, if available, will usually be enough. Occasionally a patient who is confused or agitated is in danger of injury by pulling out tubes or moving an arm with an intravenous catheter in it. Ask the family members to watch such patients and stop them hurting themselves. Tell them to call for help if necessary. Sometimes you may need to restrict the patient's movements with a restraint. Always use the least restrictive device possible.

Take all precautions to prevent the spread of infection. Keep the patient clean, keep the bedclothes clean, keep all surfaces clean, keep the floor clean, and keep the toilet clean. Make sure air is circulating. Do not allow wet dirty clothes or linens to stay in the patient's room. Help the family to understand the importance of cleanliness in preventing infection.

 ## Show families how to help with patient care

Family members are often willing to help care for the patient if they are allowed to do so. Show them how to provide care in the following ways:

- Tell family members always to wash their hands before giving care.

- Teach family members how to turn the patient so that they do not hurt him or her.

- Instruct the family on how to bathe the patient and how to give mouth care, hair care and foot care.

- Show a family member how to give the patient a back rub.

- Show the family how to do range of motion exercises and how to help the patient to get up and sit in a chair or walk.

- Tell the family what the patient can eat, and teach them about food preparation. Show them how to help the patient eat and how to encourage him or her to drink fluids.

- Show the family how to help the patient to the bathroom and, if intake and output are being measured, how to make a note about the number of times the patient urinates.

- Tell the family to keep a careful eye on the patient and report anything that might signal a problem.

5 Protect the patient from infection

An important responsibility of the nurse is to prevent the spread of infection in hospitals. Many people in hospital carry infections. Patients can be infected by these germs (microorganisms). They are carried by staff who have not properly washed their hands or whose uniforms are contaminated, by dust or droplets of air carrying infection, by visitors with disease, by other patients with disease, or by equipment or materials that are not sterile. Because they are already sick or have recently had surgery, patients can become infected very easily. Preventing the spread of infections is extremely important in hospitals.

Prevent infection

The easiest way to prevent the spread of infection is to destroy the germs when they are on hands, equipment and furniture, such as patient beds. Effective ways to destroy germs include:

- Antisepsis - destroys or stops the growth of germs.

- Decontamination - makes objects safer to handle before cleaning.

- Cleaning - removes dirt and germs from skin and objects, using soap and water.

- High-level disinfection - destroys most germs on objects.

- Sterilization - destroys all germs on objects, such as surgical instruments.

Additional methods to prevent infection include:

- Protective clothing
- Safe disposal of bodily wastes and infected articles, such as dressings.

To prevent the spread of infection in hospitals, nurses and other health care providers follow the practices of medical and surgical asepsis.

Clean technique (medical asepsis) reduces the number of germs present and prevents them from being passed on to patients.

Surgical technique (surgical asepsis) involves keeping objects and areas free of germs to make sure that procedures are sterile.

Clean technique

For clean technique, follow these guidelines:

- Clean wounds outward from the wound site. Change soiled dressings or bandages and properly dispose of them. Use normal saline to wash wounds that are clean. Use Betadine and Chlorhexidine to clean the skin. Use a soap and water wash for dirty wounds.

- Prevent the spread of microorganisms in droplets. Encourage patients to cover their mouth with tissue or a handkerchief when coughing or sneezing.

- Never have patients share personal items. Keep the bedside clean and dry. It should not have water and open bottles of solution on it.

- Clean and disinfect soiled reusable objects.

- Do not let soiled linens and other articles touch your uniform. Dispose of them appropriately.

- Empty suction and drainage bottles before they become full.

- Do not raise dust by shaking linens.

- Never put supplies or equipment on the floor.

- Wear clean disposable gloves, if available, when handling body fluids. Wash your hands after taking off the gloves.

- Wear a protective gown or apron, if available, whenever you are carrying out a "dirty" procedure.

- When a patient area is dirty, first clean the area that is the least soiled. Clean the most soiled area last.

- Pour liquids into the sink close to the drain so that they do not splash.

- Put used disposable needles and syringes and other "sharps" in puncture-resistant containers for disposal.

- Wash your hands frequently.

    - Wash hands before and after eating, preparing food or feeding.

    - Wash hands after using the toilet.

    - Wash hands after blowing your nose, coughing or sneezing into your hands.

> **Wash your hands before and after contact with a patient.**

    - Wash hands before and after special nursing procedures.

    - Wash hands before and after contact with wounds.

- ◆ Wash hands after handling soiled linens and waste.

- ◆ Wash hands before and after wearing gloves.

- ◆ Wash hands after contact with a patient.

- ◆ Wash hands after handling contaminated dressings or equipment such as a bedpan.

Hand-washing technique

Thorough hand washing is the most effective way to prevent the spread of infection in hospitals. These principles are important for effective hand washing:

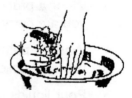

- Always remove jewellery before washing hands.

- Use soap and running water, if available.

- Wet your hands and wrists, keeping hands lower than the elbows. This allows water to flow to your fingertips and avoids contaminating your arms.

- Lather thoroughly. Use firm rubbing and circular motions for 30 seconds to wash the palms, back of the hands, fingers, between the fingers, knuckles, wrists and forearms.

- If your hands are visibly soiled, scrub them for one to four minutes.

- Clean under your fingernails.

- If you use bar soap, after washing, rinse the soap with water.

- If there is running water, rinse your hands thoroughly. Use a pitcher if there is no running water. Do not dip your hands into a bowl to rinse. This will recontaminate them.

> **Avoid repeatedly dipping your hands into a basin of water, even when an antiseptic has been added.**

- Dry your hands carefully with a clean dry towel or air dry them.

- Use a corner of the clean towel to turn off the water if the tap (faucet) is hand operated, not operated by foot or elbow.

It is the nurse's responsibility to try to make sure that every patient has a container for water, soap and a clean towel. When no running water is available, use one of the following:

> *Clinical alert:*
> **Wash your hands frequently even if running water is not available.**

- a bucket with a tap which can be turned on and off

- a bucket and pitcher

If you use a bucket of fresh water, always empty it and fill it again with fresh water for the next person to use.

Care of equipment

Cleaning is also necessary for objects used in patient care.

Before washing used surgical instruments, re-usable needles and syringes, and gloves, they should be decontaminated. 0.5% chlorine bleach solution is best to use for decontamination because it quickly kills the HIV/AIDS and hepatitis B virus. However, 0.5% chlorine bleach solution quickly loses its power to kill germs. Prepare a fresh solution every day. Change it as soon as it looks dirty. It is also good for cleaning blood spills. If you do not have chlorine bleach, alcohol or a phenolic solution may be used.

When you are washing soiled objects, first rinse them with cold water to get off organic material such as mucus and blood. Then wash the article in hot soapy water. Use a brush to clean grooves and corners that are hard to get at. Finally, rinse off the soap and dry them.

To disinfect objects, use a chemical preparation (disinfectant) such as phenol or iodine compounds. Disinfection with sodium and calcium hypochlorite, for example, destroys existing germs on objects but will not kill spores, viruses or fungi. Antiseptics are less concentrated than disinfectants. Antiseptics are used for hands or other skin areas. They include iodine, alcohol, Chlorhexidine, and Betadine.

Sterilization, or the destruction of all microorganisms, can be done by physical (steam under pressure, using an autoclave or pressure cooker), or chemical means. Dry heat is a less reliable sterilization process than wet sterilization (steam under pressure). Boiling in water, if carefully carried out, can provide **high-level disinfection, not sterilization.**

 Sterile technique

Sterile techniques (surgical asepsis) are used in the operating room and the delivery room. You should also use sterile techniques at the patient's bedside for invasive procedures:

- inserting an intravenous needle
- suctioning the patient's airway

- inserting a urinary catheter

- changing wound dressings.

Clinical alert: **Always use sterile techniques when doing a procedure that could introduce infection into the patient's body. Protect the patient as well as possible against infection.**

Surgical technique needs a work area with no microorganisms (a sterile field). This area contains sterile items for surgery or other invasive procedures:

A sterile field is usually a sterile drape or a thick layer of waxed paper or the opened package in which sterile items were packed. The sterile field is put on a clean, cold, smooth, dry working surface such as a cart. (A cart used for aseptic techniques should not be used for other purposes.) Sterile techniques are used to stop germs going into the body and to prevent the spread of infection. These are the basic principles of sterile technique:

- Wash your hands thoroughly. Rub your hands with a bactericidal solution such as Chlorhexidine, if available.

- Keep your hands higher than your elbows while washing. This stops any contaminants on your forearm from reaching your hands.

- Put on sterile gloves if doing procedures at the bedside. In the operating room, also put on a sterile gown and a surgical cap, and wear a mask.

- Sterile objects become unsterile if they are touched by an unsterile object, or if they are out of vision, or below the waist of the nurse.

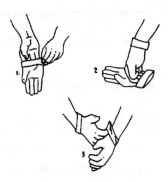

Putting on sterile gloves

Any object that becomes unsterile must be resterilized before it is used.

- Moving air can carry microorganisms. Keep doors closed and traffic to a minimum where a sterile procedure is being performed.

- Make sure that windows are screened or closed and strict rodent control is maintained in the operating theatre/suite.

> *Clinical alert:* **If there is any question about sterility, assume the object is unsterile.**

- Do not sneeze or cough over a sterile field. Talk as little as possible.

Universal precautions

Universal precautions are recommended for blood and for all body fluids, and excretions. They are to prevent the spread of blood-borne pathogens. These include hepatitis B virus, hepatitis C virus, and human immunodeficiency virus (HIV).

Follow the universal precautions with all patients.

- The most important universal precaution is hand-washing. Immediately wash your hands and any other skin surfaces that are contaminated with blood, body fluids containing blood, or other potentially infectious body fluids.

- Be extremely careful with sharp objects. Use one hand to recap a clean needle. Place the cap on a flat surface and slide the needle in. Do not recap needles which will be disposed of. Do not remove used needles from disposable syringes by hand. Do not bend, break or otherwise move used needles by hand.

- To prevent needlestick injuries, put used disposable syringes and needles, scalpel blades and other sharp items in puncture-resistant containers for disposal immediately after use. Keep these containers as close as possible to where sharp objects will be used.

- Take care to avoid injuries when using needles, scalpels and other sharp instruments, cleaning used instruments and disposing of used needles and sharps.

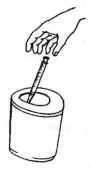

Throw away sharp objects in puncture-resistant containers

- When possible, protect yourself when you are exposed to blood and other fluids that could infect you. Wear gloves when you are in contact with blood or other body fluids containing blood. Change your gloves after patient contact. Wear gowns in situations where it is likely that droplets of blood or body fluids will be sprayed. Wear a mask and goggles when droplets of blood or other body fluids may spray onto your eyes, nose or mouth. Use a mouthpiece or resuscitation bag when providing resuscitation.

- Handle soiled linen as little as possible. Put linen which is soiled with blood or body fluids in leak-resistant bags. Put all specimens of blood and body fluids in containers with secure lids. Get rid of infective waste following hospital policy.

- Use a disinfectant to decontaminate work surfaces when there is a spill of blood or other body fluids. If there is not very much disinfectant, do not dilute the solutions, because that makes them ineffective.

- Do not care for a patient when you have open skin lesions. If you must do so, wear gloves.

 # Gloves

Wear latex gloves if you are likely to touch blood or body fluids. If there are not many gloves, keep them for when they are most needed, for example, when you expect a lot of contact with blood. If you are going to re-use gloves, look at them carefully and get rid of damaged ones. To examine them for damage, gently blow the gloves full of air, twist the cuff and hold them under clean water. You could also fill them with clean water and squeeze them to see if they leak. Wash off any blood and body fluids from gloves which are undamaged. Use water, but not soap, and disinfect them. Finally, sterilize the gloves. Good quality latex gloves can be boiled or bleached five or more times. Dry the gloves away from direct sunlight.

 # Isolation technique

You may sometimes need to isolate a patient to prevent the spread of infection. This can happen when a patient has a disease which is easily caught by others (a highly contagious or highly virulent disease) or an infection that is resistant to standard antibiotics. The aim of isolation is to protect other patients in the hospital, visitors and staff, while also giving the right care to the infected patient.

Ideally, put the contagious person in a separate room with the door closed. Anyone entering the room should wear a gown, mask and gloves, if available. Maintain a strict control of visitors. Put a sign on the door to inform anyone entering that this person is in isolation.

Do not avoid the patient who is in isolation. Give the patient who has a contagious disease the same kind, respectful treatment that is given to other patients.

If a patient is to be isolated, prepare the room by getting rid of all unnecessary furniture. The patient should also have as few things as possible in the room. All these things should be washable. Store everything the patient will need in the room to prevent unnecessary coming and going.

Dishes used by the patient must be washed separately. The patient should have a separate toilet or separate bedpan and urinal. Wash these separately.

Put contaminated articles from the patient's room in a plastic-lined container or bag. Label this as infectious. Keep a sharps container in the room. Dispose of urine, faeces, and vomit at once. Mop up any spilled fluids immediately and clean the area with disinfectant. Make sure that cleaning staff understand the restrictions. Use separate cleaning equipment for this room. When in the room, cleaning staff should wear gloves if available.

After any contact with the patient, remove your gloves and wash your hands with antiseptic solution or soap and water.

Patient education

Carefully explain to the patient and family why restrictions are necessary. Make sure that the person does not feel emotionally isolated or viewed as somehow bad. The patient and family are much more likely to cooperate with the restrictions if they understand them but do not feel accused. Let them ask questions and discuss their fears.

Patients who need strict isolation can develop problems. They can feel stigmatized. They are alone all the time and do not have any stimulation. Be alert for the problems that may come up, such as high anxiety and confusion, resulting from too little stimulation. Try to talk with the patient regularly. Bring the patient a radio or reading materials. Above all, be courteous and accepting. Do not convey any feelings of disgust or fear about the infection.

 # How to care for the patient with a contagious disease

Patients with tuberculosis

Patients with pulmonary tuberculosis (TB) should be put in private rooms or a separate ward. If a separate ward is not available, keep them in a part of the ward away from other patients. A suspected TB patient should not be put in a TB ward until you know that he or she definitely has the disease. Patients who are HIV positive should never be in contact with TB patients since they are especially vulnerable to TB infection.

TB patient rooms should be well ventilated. The doors should be closed to the hall and the windows open to the outside. This will reduce the chance of airborne infection. If possible, patient rooms should have large uncurtained windows to let in sunlight.

Do not dry sweep the room or shake out soiled bedding and clothing indoors. The infection may be spread through particles on dust from bedding, dressings, floors, etc. Soiled bedding and clothes should be washed immediately.

A face mask reduces the risk of infecting others. TB patients and those suspected of having TB should wear a mask when moving from one part of the hospital to another and during procedures. The patient could use a clean handkerchief or a cloth tied over the nose and mouth. This will protect other patients and the nurses. It is not helpful for the nurse to wear a mask unless she is doing a procedure that induces a cough. Visiting family members should not wear masks.

Hand-washing after contact with the patient is absolutely essential.

The best way to prevent the spread of TB is by rapid diagnosis and treatment of infectious cases. All patients with tuberculosis should be on short-course chemotherapy for the disease. Infectious patients usually become non-infectious within about two to four weeks, and symptoms improve. The risk to others stops.

An infant should be separated from an infectious mother for two to four weeks; after that she will not be contagious. If the mother is taking the medicine, she can still breast-feed. During the time when she is separated from the infant, she should hand express the breast milk to ensure that she will have breast milk after the two to four weeks.

It is essential that patients take every single dose of the drug prescribed. Teach patients and the family that TB is curable as long as the patient takes regularly the whole course of medicine prescribed. The course of treatment usually lasts six to nine months. To ensure that patients take their medications regularly, direct supervision by a health worker is required for at least the first two months of treatment.

Explain to patients that if they stop taking the drug, they risk developing drug-resistant TB. They will also become infectious again, putting others at risk. Show patients how to reduce the risk of infecting others, by covering their mouth with their hand when coughing and using a sputum pot with a lid. Tell the patient and family to avoid spitting. Above all, be kind to the patients and do not avoid them because of the disease.

Leprosy patients

Few leprosy patients are hospitalized. Treatment is generally on an outpatient basis. Within one week of beginning the standard multiple drug therapy, leprosy patients are not contagious. It is important to understand this if you have leprosy patients in your hospital. No precautions need to be taken to protect other patients or staff. There is also no risk for the baby of a mother with leprosy.

Children who receive the BCG vaccine for tuberculosis are also protected against leprosy.

When you care for patients with leprosy, do not make the patients feel that they are bad because they have the disease, as was done in the past. This is important. You can help the patient to understand the importance of taking the medicines regularly and completely to be cured. For patients at risk of nerve damage, teach simple protection. For example, the person should wear shoes to protect insensitive feet, use gloves when working with hot or sharp objects, and use goggles to protect his or her eyes against dust.

Teach the patient to soak his or her hands and apply Vaseline regularly to prevent cracks. If the person has stiff joints, teach him or her to do range of motion exercises. If there are cracks on the patient's feet, he or she should also soak the feet and apply Vaseline.

Patients with Human Immunodeficiency Virus (HIV) and Acquired Immune Deficiency Syndrome (AIDS)

The human immunodeficiency virus (HIV), which is the virus that causes acquired immune deficiency syndrome or AIDS, can be transmitted through:

- unprotected vaginal or anal intercourse
- any unprotected contact with blood, semen, or vaginal fluids
- blood transfusions or blood products obtained from donors
- from mother to infant during pregnancy or labour or through breast-feeding.

The AIDS virus is extremely dangerous, but it is also very fragile and dies quickly. It cannot be spread by any casual contact or by coughing, sneezing or touching, by sharing dishes or cups or by food or water. The most common way of spreading the infection is through sexual intercourse.

A person infected with the virus may have no symptoms of disease for years but can infect others.

Most people with HIV will eventually develop acquired immune-deficiency syndrome or AIDS. Symptoms include:

- very reduced immunity to other diseases

- unexplained persistent night sweats

- fatigue

- weight loss

- enlarged lymph glands

- persistent diarrhoea

- skin rashes or bluish-purple skin lesions

- thick grey-white coating on the tongue, mucous membranes or throat

- chronic cough and recurrent lung or other body infections.

- opportunistic infections: these are infections from microorganisms that are commonly found in the body but do not cause problems if the immune system is functioning properly.

Care of the patient with AIDS requires universal precautions, just as for patients with other blood-borne pathogens. The risk of infection of health care workers is extremely low if the universal precautions listed earlier in this chapter are followed. Since AIDS is fatal, these precautions are essential.

Blood is the most likely route for the virus to be passed on (transmitted) in hospitals. This happens through a needlestick injury or through injury with another sharp instrument contaminated with the blood of the infected person. The virus is not passed on through unbroken skin. It can be passed on if open sores are exposed to infected blood or other body fluids. It can also be passed on through splashes of infected blood onto mucous membranes.

To prevent transmission of the virus, be especially careful with disposable needles and other sharp instruments. Use them only once and put them into a sharps container immediately after use. Then burn or bury them. Wear thick gloves to clean any reusable sharp instruments, then disinfect or sterilize them.

Many people are living longer with the disease today. It is important to teach AIDS patients and their families to take care of the patient at home and avoid problems. Good nutrition and enough rest and sleep are especially important. Also, the patient should stay as active as possible. Exercise is good. However, patients should avoid unnecessary exposure to other infections.

Tell the family that it is safe to care for the person with AIDS. They should wash their hands with soap and water after changing soiled bed sheets or after contact with body fluids. If clothing or sheets are stained with blood or diarrhoea, keep them separate from other washing. First rinse the stain off, holding the cloth by an unstained part. Then wash as normal. Also, keep bed clothes clean. If a family member has open wounds, they should be covered and someone else should wash the patient's clothes and bedding. Do not share toothbrushes, razors, or needles. Finally, to avoid giving other infections to the person with AIDS, wash hands before cooking, eating, feeding another person or giving medicine.

Patients with other contagious diseases

Patients with hepatitis A, typhoid fever, cholera and encephalitis need to be in a separate room only if they cannot control their urine (they are incontinent). Patients with meningitis need to be isolated only for the first 24 hours. Wear a gown or protective apron if available. Wear gloves if you are touching infected material. It is essential to wash your hands after contact with the patient.

6 Safe administration of medicines

It is the nurse's responsibility safely to prepare and give the drugs ordered by the doctor. If not given properly, medicines can be harmful or even fatal. Before giving any medication the nurse needs to know:

- the doses of the drug which are safe to administer
- the dose of the drug which has been prescribed for the patient
- the method of administration
- the drug's actions and expected effects
- possible side effects (unintended effects).

It is also important to know if a patient is allergic to a drug. Ask your patients about any bad reactions they have had to drugs in the past.

> **Five rights of drug administration:**
> ◊ right dose
> ◊ right drug
> ◊ right patient
> ◊ right route
> ◊ right time

For safe administration of drugs: give the right dose of the right drug to the right patient in the right route at the right time.

When giving medications, the nurse needs to be aware of possible interactions between the patient's different drugs. Drug interactions can sometimes harm the patient.

It is the nurse's responsibility to protect the patient from harm. If you think the wrong drug or the wrong dose has been ordered, ask for help from the nurse or the doctor in charge.

Right dose

The nurse needs to know the doses of the drug which are safe to administer. Sometimes the pharmacy gives out drugs in grams when the order specifies milligrams, or the other way around. You need to convert these. Remember that:

> **1000 mg (milligrams) = 1 g (gram)**
>
> **1000 g = 1 kg (kilogram)**
>
> **1000 ml (millilitre) = 1 l (litre)**

Liquid medicines

Sometimes liquid medicines are given in a vial or an ampoule. A vial is a glass or plastic bottle that may hold one or more doses of a drug. An ampoule is a small sterile plastic or glass container that holds one dose of a drug. Usually it has a small neck with a coloured mark to show where the neck can easily be snapped off and the drug drawn out .

Sometimes the vial may contain more than the dose you need to give. You need then to work out how much of the solution to give in order to have the correct dose.

You can calculate using this formula:

$$\frac{\text{Dose you want (mg)}}{\text{Dose on hand}} \quad x \quad \text{volume on hand} = \text{amount (volume in ml) needed to give}$$

Thus, if you need to give a dose of 500 mg of ampicillin and it is in a solution containing 250 mg in 5 ml, you would work out this formula:

$$\frac{500}{250} \text{ x 5 ml } = 10 \text{ ml}$$

The correct dose would be 10 ml.

Pills or capsules

If the drug is in pills or capsules, look at the container to see how much of the drug is in each pill. If the drug is not separately packaged in the amount you need, calculate the amount to use. The correct number of pills is the desired dose divided by the amount of drug in each pill.

If you need to give 100 mg of the drug, and each pill in the bottle has 50 mg, then you need to give the patient two pills. Sometimes you have to calculate a fractional or smaller dose, particularly when giving a drug to a child. Adult dosages of most drugs are standard, but children's doses are not standard. A child's dose is normally based on his or her body weight in kilograms.

Right route

There are several routes for administration of drugs:.

- **by mouth** (orally), in pills, capsules or liquids
- **by injection** (parenterally), into the body tissues by a needle and syringe
- **on a certain area** (topically), applied to the skin or mucous membranes
- **in the eye or ear**
- **into the rectum** (rectally), in suppositories or by inserting some fluid.

Always make sure that you are using the right route.

Right drug

To make sure that you give the right patient the right drug, check what you are doing at every step.

Guidelines for administering medication:

- Check the patient's medication card or record against the doctor's order. Make sure that what is on the card is what the doctor ordered.

- Compare the label on the medicine bottle or package wrap with the patient's medication card or record. Make sure that you have the right medicine.

- After you have prepared the medication, recheck the label before taking the medicine to the patient's room.

Right patient

Make sure you give the right medication to the right patient. Many patients have similar last names. Therefore you must:

- check the medication card/record against the patient's name on the bed or other patient identification

- ask the patient to tell you his or her name.

Right time

Many drugs are ordered for certain times of the day. Insulin, for example, is normally given before meals. Antibiotics are usually ordered every 6, 8 or 12 hours, throughout the day and night (around the clock), not just during waking hours. They must be given around the clock to maintain high enough levels of the drug in the patient's body. Diuretics are usually given in the morning rather than the evening, so that the patient's sleep is not disturbed by frequent urination. Know the medication schedule your hospital or institution uses and give drugs at the scheduled times.

Giving oral medication

The easiest, safest and most convenient way to give medication is through the mouth. If you know that it is difficult for the patient to swallow, you can crush tablets into a powder. Then mix the powder with some soft food that the patient can swallow. Not all drugs can be crushed. For example, drugs with a protective coating or those in a slow release form should not be crushed.

Wash your hands. Calculate the amount you need. Take the liquid or solid medicine to the patient's room on a cart or tray, and make sure that you have the right person.

If you are giving any medicines that require you to assess the patient, do that first. If the vital signs indicate problems, check with the doctor or the nurse in charge before giving the drug.

Clinical alert: **Drugs that require you to check vital signs include:**

- **digoxin--check pulse**
- **hypotensive drugs (drugs that reduce blood pressure)--check blood pressure**
- **narcotics--check breathing.**

If this is the first time the patient is getting a medication, explain what the drug is for. If it has side effects, tell the patient what to expect.

Help the patient to sit up or lie on one side. This makes it easier to swallow the medicine.

If the patient says that this medicine is not the same as he or she was given before, check the order again to make sure that it is correct.

Give liquid medicine in a cup to the patient to swallow. If the patient cannot hold the cup, bring it to his or her mouth. If the medicine has an unpleasant taste, give the patient some juice or bread with the medicine to cover its taste.

Give a glass of water to the patient with the pills. This will help the patient to swallow. If he or she cannot hold the cup, you should hold it, and give one pill at a time, followed by a sip of water.

> *Clinical alert:* **Stay with the patient until he or she has swallowed all the medicines.**

Always go back and check the patient for any adverse reactions or side effects from the medication.

Write down the medication the patient has taken. Give the name of the drug, dose, method of administration, time of administration and any important patient information such as the pulse rate.

Oral medication for children

Many medications are given to children in a dropper, a syringe or cup. It is important to measure small amounts of medicine accurately. For volumes less than 1 ml, use a tuberculin syringe, if one is available, or other syringe, with no needle attached. You can put the medication directly into the child's mouth from the syringe, or pour it from a small cup.

Young children and some older children have trouble swallowing pills. If a liquid preparation is not available, crush the tablets and mix them with soft food.

Give medication to children while they are sitting up, so that they do not choke on it.

> *Clinical alert*: **The safest and cheapest way to give medicine is by mouth.**

Injecting medication

Medicine may be injected (given parenterally) into the skin, under the skin, into a muscle, or into a vein. Drugs given in any of these ways are absorbed more quickly than drugs taken by mouth. Therefore it is especially important to be sure that you give the right drug to the right person in the right amount.

To give medicines parenterally, the nurse uses a vial or ampoule, a syringe and a needle. A syringe has three parts: the tip connecting with the needle; the outside or barrel, on which a scale is printed, usually in millilitres, to indicate how much is in the syringe; and the plunger, which fits inside the barrel and is used to push the drug up into the needle. Re-usable glass syringes and disposable plastic syringes are used in many hospitals and clinics. The plastic syringes are usually in individual packages to make sure they are sterile. They may come already filled with a unit dose.

> *Clinical alert:* **Plastic syringes must be thrown away after use to prevent the spread of infection.**

There are different sizes of syringes for different uses. The most common types are the hypodermic syringe (which is used to give medication), the insulin syringe and the tuberculin syringe. The insulin syringe is like the hypodermic syringe but it has a special scale on the side that shows the amount of insulin inside. The tuberculin syringe is narrow and is marked (calibrated) in tenths and hundredths of a millilitre. This type of syringe is useful for giving very small doses.

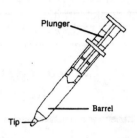

The three parts of a syringe

The needle also has three parts: the hub, which fits onto the syringe; the thin shaft fastened to the hub; and the bevel, which is the slanted part at the tip. Needles may be shorter or longer, with larger or smaller diameters (gauges) and smaller or longer slants. The gauge may vary from #14 to #28. The one with the largest diameter is #14 and #28 is the smallest.

Needles with longer bevels are sharper and are less uncomfortable for the patient. For injections under the skin, use a short needle with a small diameter and long bevel.

For injections into the muscle, use a longer needle with a larger diameter and a long bevel. Use a short bevel for injections into the skin or into a vein. Children and small adults usually need shorter needles. Assess the patient to decide on the right size. All packaged needles come with a cap.

> *Clinical alert:* **Never leave a needle in a vial.**

Injections into the skin

An intradermal injection is given in the dermal layer of the skin, just below the top layer, which is called the epidermis. Intradermal injections are used for allergy tests, tuberculin tests, and many immunizations. The most common site for

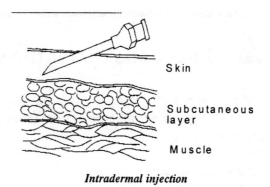

Intradermal injection

this type of injection is the lower arm. Other sites include the upper chest and the back beneath the shoulder blade. BCG vaccination is also given intradermally. The most common sites are the upper arm, forearm and buttocks or upper thigh. To give a BCG injection or other intradermal injection:

- Wash your hands before you begin.

- Check the name of the patient.

- Tell the patient that the injection will cause a small lump, like a mosquito bite or small blister, but it will disappear quickly. Select a site that has no discoloration or rash or broken skin. Clean the site with alcohol if you have it, or another cleansing agent, using a circular motion.

- Pull the patient's skin flat. Hold the syringe at about a 15° angle, and insert the needle through the epidermis into the dermis.

- Inject the fluid slowly until a lump appears. This indicates that the fluid is in the dermis.

- Take the needle out quickly and lightly wipe the site with an antiseptic swab or cotton ball.

Clinical alert: **Do not massage the injection site because that might make the medication go into the tissue or out of the injection site.**

 ## Injections under the skin

Subcutaneous injections go into the fatty tissue just below the skin. Many drugs are injected subcutaneously, including vaccines, preoperative medications, narcotics, insulin and heparin. Common sites for subcutaneous injections are: the backs of the upper arms and the fronts of the thighs, the upper back, and the fat pads on the abdomen.

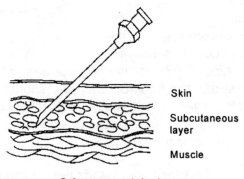

Skin

Subcutaneous layer

Muscle

Subcutaneous injection

- Wash your hands.

- Before giving the medicine, check the patient's name.

- Draw the medication into the syringe.

- Get rid of any air bubbles in the syringe by tipping the syringe upside down and slowly pushing the plunger until you can see a drop of solution in the needle's bevel or end.

- Grasp the patient's skin with the thumb and forefinger of your left hand (right if you are left-handed) to raise up the subcutaneous tissue and form a fat fold.

- With your right hand, put the needle in at a 45° or 90° angle and pull slowly back on the plunger to see whether you have entered a blood vessel.

Clinical alert: **If blood comes into the syringe when you pull back the plunger, you have hit a vein. Then you must withdraw the needle, discard the syringe and prepare a new injection. That is because subcutaneous injections can be dangerous if they go directly into the bloodstream, where they are absorbed more quickly than from the fatty tissue.**

- If no blood comes into the syringe, give the injection by slowly and steadily pushing the plunger.

- Quickly take the needle out and press down on the skin.

- There is usually no bleeding from subcutaneous injections. However, if there is bleeding, press gently until it stops.

 ## Injections into the muscle

Intramuscular injections (that is, injections into the muscle) are absorbed faster than subcutaneous injections. Large injections (up to 1-2 ml for a child and 3 ml

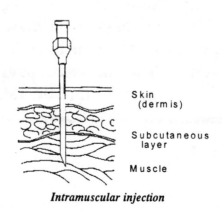

Skin (dermis)

Subcutaneous layer

Muscle

Intramuscular injection

for an adult) can be given this way because muscle can absorb more fluid than fatty tissues.

The preferred sites for intramuscular injections are the dorsogluteal site in the gluteus medius muscle in the posterior hip or the ventrogluteal site in the gluteus medius muscle in the lateral hip (see below).

Ventrogluteal site

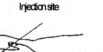

The ventrogluteal injection site is easy to identify and safe to use. It avoids major nerves and blood vessels.

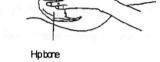

Ventrogluteal site for intramuscular injection

Dorsogluteal site

If you use the dorsogluteal site, you must be careful to avoid the sciatic nerve, because accidental injection into this nerve can cause permanent or partial paralysis of the leg.

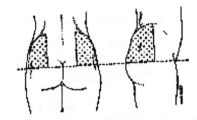

Dorsogluteal site for intramuscular injection

Clinical alert: **Never use the dorsogluteal site in the posterior hip for infants or children who have not yet begun to walk. Give the injection in the rectus femoris muscle or the vastus lateralis site in the middle third of the thigh.**

Intramuscular injection sites for infants and small children

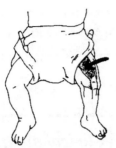

Rectus femoris site for intramuscular injection

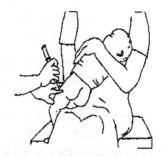

Giving intramuscular injection to child. Vastus lateralis site for intramuscular injection

Deltoid muscle

The muscle of the upper arm, the deltoid muscle, can also be used for an older child or an adult. However, remember that you cannot inject as much fluid into the arm as into the muscles of the hip.

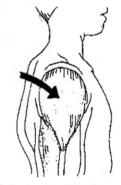

Injection into deltoid muscle

How to give injections into the muscle

- Wash your hands.

- Protect the patient's privacy by putting a sheet over body parts that do not need to be exposed.

- If you are giving an injection to a child, show the mother how to hold the child.

- Choose a site for the injection that has no broken skin, swelling, hardness, tenderness, redness or warmth. Locate the exact site and clean it

> *Clinical alert:* **Do not inject more than 1 ml into the arm of an adult or a child.**

with an antiseptic swab or cotton ball using a circular motion and extending outward about 5 cm on each side or 10 cm in total.

- Using your left hand, stretch the skin at the site. This makes it firmer so that it is easier to insert the needle.

- Insert the needle quickly at a 90° angle through the skin and into the muscle.

- Aspirate by pulling back on the plunger. If blood appears in the syringe, pull out the needle, throw away the syringe and prepare a new injection.

> *Clinical alert:* **Do not let the injection go into a blood vessel.**

- If blood does not appear, then slowly, steadily push the plunger to inject the medication.

- Quickly remove the needle and apply firm pressure to the site using an antiseptic swab.

- Wash your hands.

✔ Intravenous therapy (drip)

Intravenous therapy is putting a sterile fluid through a needle directly into the patient's vein. Usually the sterile fluid contains electrolytes (sodium, calcium, potassium), nutrients (usually glucose), vitamins or drugs.

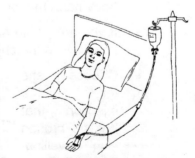

Intravenous therapy

Intravenous (IV) therapy is used to give fluids when the patient cannot swallow, is unconscious, is dehydrated or is in shock, to provide salts needed to maintain a balance of electrolytes, or glucose needed for metabolism, or to give medication.

Drugs given intravenously enter the bloodstream directly and are absorbed faster than any other kind of medication. Therefore, drugs are given in this way when a rapid effect is needed, or when the drug is too irritating to body tissues to be given any other way. Drugs given in this way are usually put in (infused) slowly to prevent reactions.

Guidelines for intravenous therapy

- Know the fluid or drug that is ordered, its actions and side effects
- Know the amount of fluid or drug to be given over what period of time
- Know the amount and type of solution in which drugs can be diluted
- Know how long a drug can be safely administered
- Know the compatibilities of all the drugs the patient is receiving
- Monitor carefully both the patient and the rate of infusion

---

 ## How to give intravenous fluids and drugs safely

You must take special care to avoid errors in calculating doses and in preparing drugs, because intravenous drugs take effect immediately. Double check the five "rights" of drug administration: right dose, right drug, right patient, right route, right time.

You must also know the desired action and potential side effects of all the intravenous drugs you give.

- Most drugs require a minimum dilution and/or rate of flow.

- Many drugs are very irritating or damaging to tissues outside the veins.

- Only one antibiotic is given at a time intravenously. The IV line is washed out (flushed) between antibiotics.

- Never give medications, sterile water, or dextrose water with blood or blood products.

- You must carefully monitor all patients on IV therapy. Watch the patient for any signs of an adverse reaction, including a rash, trouble with breathing, increased pulse rate, vomiting, and signs of dehydration or fluid overload (for these last two signs see the chapter on caring for the patient who has problems with elimination).

- Check the insertion site for swelling, redness, hardness, pain or warmth.

- Check the IV flow rate to make sure it is correct. The flow rate must be monitored extremely carefully and frequently in infants, children, the elderly, acutely ill patients and patients with dehydration, heart or kidney disease or diabetes.

How to determine how fast the IV fluid should be going in:

- First work out the drop rate of the IV tubing. A macrodrip tube can deliver 10 or 15 drops per 1 ml. Microdrip tubing delivers 60 drops per 1 ml. The number of drops required for 1 ml is called the drop factor.
- Work out the number of millilitres of fluid to administer in an hour. Divide the total amount of solution to be delivered by the number of hours the infusion will last. Then multiply that figure by the drop factor.
- To determine how many drops to administer per minute, divide by 60.
- Count the number of drops per minute that are being infused. If that is not the correct flow rate, adjust the drip rate.

Starting intravenous therapy

The site for venepuncture (inserting the needle into the vein) is usually one of the veins of the forearm or hand. Patients requiring faster running infusions or blood transfusions require larger needles and therefore larger veins.

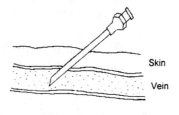

Intravenous injection

- Starting IV therapy requires sterile technique.

- Pick a vein that is easy to feel and that is fairly straight. The vein should be full, soft, and easy to feel. It should not feel hard or rubbery. Avoid veins that are inflamed (red and warm), irritated or painful.

- Try not to use a vein that has been used before, because it may be damaged.

How to add medication to an IV line

Intravenous medication can be given slowly from a bottle or bag containing a solution. This is called a continuous infusion and is similar to other intravenous therapy. Alternatively, the drug can be given all at once, and this is called an intravenous push or bolus. For a continuous infusion, the drug can be added to a new fluid container before it is hung or added to a container that is already running.

- Carefully check the medication order against the patient's medication card or record, just as you would for other routes of administration. Also make sure that the medication is compatible with the solution it is to be mixed with.

- Put the patient's name on the container with the name and amount of the drug, the flow rate, the time infusion begins, and your name or initials.

- Always check the patient to be sure that there is no adverse reaction to the drug being infused. Look for a change in pulse rate, chills, nausea, vomiting, headache or trouble with breathing. If the patient has a reaction, stop or slow the infusion rate and tell the doctor or the nurse in charge immediately.

- Record the name and amount of the drug, the solution to which it was added, and the time it was given.

How to give an IV push

For an intravenous push, you give the medication all at once, injecting the drug into an existing continuous infusion IV line.

- After inserting the needle, draw back the plunger to withdraw blood (to be sure the needle is in a vein).

- Inject the drug at the rate ordered. Be careful not to inject the drug too fast.

How to give a blood transfusion

Before giving a blood transfusion, send a sample of the patient's blood to the laboratory for typing and crossmatching, unless you already have clear information about this on the chart.

- When the blood arrives, make sure the patient's name, blood type and Rh factor are the same as those on the blood to be transfused. Do not give the blood if the information is not exactly the same.

- To prevent bacterial growth, transfuse the blood within 30 minutes of its arrival on the ward.

- Check the patient's vital signs before beginning.

- Make sure the drip chamber has a filter to trap clots or debris.

- Give a blood transfusion only with normal saline. Any other solution is incompatible with blood products.

- Stay with the patient for at least 15 minutes and observe him or her carefully for signs of a reaction. These signs include chills, nausea and vomiting, headache, muscle aches, difficulty with breathing, wheezing, fever, sweating, chest pain, tingling, numbness, and rapid pulse. **The sooner a reaction occurs, the more severe it is likely to be.**

- If there are any signs of reaction, stop the transfusion and notify the doctor immediately.

- If the patient shows no signs of reaction, continue the infusion. Check the vital signs 15 minutes after beginning the infusion. Then check again every 30 minutes until 1 hour after the transfusion is complete. Tell the patient to call a nurse immediately if he or she notices anything unusual.

- Record the time, the type of blood, the amount, and drip rate.

How to give eye medication or irrigate the eye

Sometimes the eye needs to be washed out, to clean it or to get rid of foreign particles. Also, medication may be given in the eye. Sterile technique should always be used to wash (irrigate) the eye or put in medication.

Irrigating the eye:

- Tell the patient what you are going to do and explain that it will not hurt.

- Ask the patient to tilt his or her head towards the side of the eye you are going to wash and place a small basin below the eye.

- Wash your hands. Using cotton balls moistened with sterile solution or saline, wipe the eyelids, working from the inner part to the outer side.

- Now separate the lids of the eye with your thumb and forefinger and gently press on the cheekbone beneath the eye to hold the eyelids apart and make a gutter.

- Hold the irrigator above the eye and direct the solution to the gutter. Work from the inner to the outer part of the eye.

- Then tell the patient to close his or her eye and move the eyeball around from time to time, to make sure the solution reaches all of the eye.

Instilling liquid medication into the eye:

- Tell the patient what you are going to do. Explain that it will not hurt, though the medicine may sting briefly.

- As the patient looks up, with the head tilted backward, gently pull the lower eyelid downward to make a gutter.

- Stand to the side of the patient as you work. He or she is less likely to blink if you are not directly in front.

- Put the correct number of drops into the gutter in the lower part of the eye, not directly onto the cornea.

Instilling ointment into the eye:

- To put ointment into the eye, ask the patient to hold his or her head back and look up.

- Discard the first amount of ointment that comes out of the tube. It is considered to be contaminated.

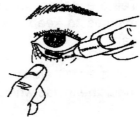

Medicine being put in the eye

- As the patient looks up, gently pull the lower eyelid downward to make a gutter.

- Hold the tube as close as possible above the eye, **without touching it,** and squeeze out 2 cm (about 1/4 the size of the fingertip) of the ointment into the gutter, working from the inner to the outer edge of the eyelid.

- Tell the patient to close the eye for two minutes but not to squeeze it shut.

When you have finished, give the patient a gauze sponge or cotton to wipe off the excess ointment on the eyelid.

How to give medication in the ear

The ear sometimes needs to be irrigated to soften earwax, remove pus, or take out a foreign object in the ear canal (see the chapter on daily care of the patient).

If the ear is inflamed or the patient feels pain there, you may need to put medicine in the ear.

- Have the patient lie on one side.

- Warm the medicine container in your hands so that the medicine will not feel cold to the patient. Then fill the ear dropper with the correct amount of medication.

- Pull the patient's earlobe up and back. Put the correct number of drops along the side of the ear canal.

- • Tell the patient to continue lying on one side for five minutes to keep the medication from going out of the ear.

  Put a small sterile cotton ball in the ear to keep the medicine inside when the patient is standing up.

7 Care for the child in hospital

When children come to the hospital, they are often seriously ill or injured. They may have life-threatening problems. Every hour without treatment makes them more likely to die. It is important for nurses to identify these children and give them priority treatment.

There should be a special area of the children's ward for emergency care and care of very sick children. It should have emergency equipment, including oxygen, ambu bags and masks, intravenous equipment and drugs. A nurse should always be available to watch over these children.

How to identify and treat children who need urgent care

NOTE: Not all guidelines for identification and treatment of children needing urgent care are the same. If these guidelines are not the same as the standard treatment guidelines of your Ministry of Health, follow the Ministry of Health guidelines.

> ## Use the ABCD signs to find which children need immediate treatment.
>
> ### Airway
> ### Breathing
> ### Circulation
> ### Neurological Danger signs

- Check the child's airway and breathing first. Look for a blockage in the mouth, throat or windpipe.

- Open the airway by gently lifting the child's jaw forward. Use suction to remove saliva or vomit. If suction is not available, wipe out the child's mouth with a damp cloth.

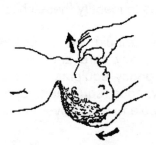

Opening the child's airway

- If the child is a blue colour (has cyanosis) or is having trouble breathing, give oxygen. Keep the airway clear.

- If the child has stopped breathing, begin mouth-to-mouth breathing immediately.

- See if the child is bleeding, and stop the bleeding.

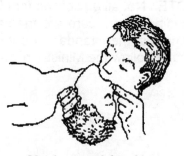

Mouth-to-mouth breathing

- Look for signs of shock: rapid, weak pulse, low blood pressure, cold and blue hands and feet, and capillary refilling time longer than two seconds.

> **How to check capillary refill time: press one of the child's fingernails between your thumb and finger until it is white, then see how long the colour takes to return.**

Pinch the child's nostrils closed with your fingers. Cover the child's mouth with your mouth and blow strongly so that the child's chest rises. Pause to let the air come back out and blow again. Repeat about once every five seconds. With babies and small children, cover the nose and mouth with your mouth and breathe **very gently** once every three seconds. Continue mouth-to-mouth breathing until the child can breathe on his or her own.

- If the child shows signs of shock, quickly give intravenous fluids. Also give oral rehydration salts (ORS) solution if the child is able to drink. Feed ORS with a spoon. Do not use a bottle.

- Put an unconscious child in the coma position.

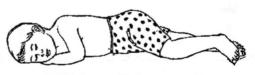

Child lying on side in coma position

- If the child is having convulsions, clear secretions with suction or a clean cloth. **Do not force an object such as a spoon or spatula into the child's mouth.**

- If the convulsions last more than five minutes or the child is cyanotic or has lowered blood pressure, give oxygen. Prepare to start treatment with diazepam (Valium). Watch closely for reduced breathing (respiratory depression).

Clinical alert: **Diazepam (Valium) is given either intravenously or rectally; it is not given by intramuscular injection.**

- Check the child's blood sugar. If it is low and the child is unconscious, prepare to give intravenous glucose. If you do not have any, insert a nasogastric tube, check that it is in the stomach. Then give 50 ml of sugar water through the nasogastric tube. **To make the sugar water, dissolve 5 gm (1 rounded teaspoon) of sugar in 50 ml (3 1/2 tablespoons) of water**. If the child is conscious, give 50 ml of sugar water by mouth. If you cannot measure blood sugar, assume the child has low blood sugar and treat it.

- Make a blood film for malaria parasites.

Continue to check the child's consciousness, using the following scale:

A=0 the child is Alert
V=1 the child responds to Voice
P=2 the child responds only to Pain
U=3 the child is Unresponsive to
**   stimulation.**

Care for children with severe diarrhoea and dehydration

The child with mild diarrhoea and no signs of dehydration is usually cared for at home. Home treatment of children with diarrhoea is discussed in the chapter on caring for the patient who has problems with elimination.

Many children come into the hospital because they have mild or severe dehydration, persistent diarrhoea, or bloody diarrhoea that shows no improvement. You must know how to assess the degree of dehydration in an infant or child quickly and to begin the right treatment.

Signs of dehydration

- general condition - restless or irritable
- thirst
- sunken eyes
- dry mouth and tongue
- rapid pulse
- poor skin elasticity (turgor). When the skin is pinched, the skinfold stays up for a few seconds instead of falling back at once

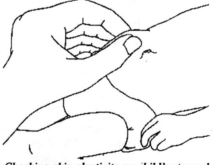

Checking skin elasticity on child's stomach

- very fast breathing and very deep breathing.

Clinical alert: **Severe dehydration needs immediate treatment. A severely dehydrated child is lethargic or unconscious or floppy. The child drinks poorly or is not able to drink at all, and the skin goes back very slowly when pinched.**

Children with severe dehydration

The prevention of dehydration is discussed in the chapter on caring for the patient who has problems with elimination. This chapter focuses on the treatment of the severely ill child.

- Children with severe dehydration should quickly be given intravenous fluids (Ringer's lactate, Hartman's solution, or, if not available, normal saline). If the child can drink, he or she should also be given oral rehydration salts (ORS) solution while the drip is being set up. If the child cannot drink, give ORS solution as soon as he or she can drink without difficulty.

Clinical alert: **If a child cannot drink and an IV line cannot be inserted, put in a nasogastric tube and give ORS solution by tube.**

- When the child is improving and can drink, stop the IV and give ORS solution. The signs of improvement include urination, improved consciousness, and more normal breathing and pulse rates (unless the child has an infection or heart failure or is overhydrated). Watch the child for several hours before discharge to be sure he or she can retain fluids.

Feeding the dehydrated child

Feeding is essential. If the child is a young infant, the mother should be encouraged to continue breast-feeding, or the infant may be given yoghurt. Older infants and children should be given food six times a day as soon as they can eat.

A child who has had diarrhoea for 14 days or more may have a serious infection. It is important to diagnose the infection and treat it with antibiotics. It is also important to give:

- the right fluids to prevent and treat dehydration

- a nutritious diet that does not make the diarrhoea worse

- supplementary vitamins and minerals because many of these children are malnourished.

Two types of diets may be especially helpful.

Diet #1: Mix together:	Diet #2: Mix together:
5 full teaspoons of cooked rice 2/5 tea cup of whole fresh milk 3/4 teaspoon oil 2/3 flat teaspoon sugar Add enough water to make a full tea cup.	1 full teaspoon cooked rice 2 small eggs or 1 1/2 full teaspoons mashed or ground chicken or fish 1 teaspoon oil 2/3 flat teaspoon of sugar Add enough water to make up to a full tea cup. Cook if using raw eggs.

- For either diet, give one full tea cup for each kilogram of body weight each day for seven days. If the child responds to the diet, add fresh fruit and well cooked vegetables. Then move to a regular diet, including milk.

- Do not give antibiotics for diarrhoea unless it is caused by an intestinal infection (shigellosis, amoebiasis or giardiasis).

- Bloody diarrhoea (dysentery) is usually caused by the shigella bacteria. Children should be treated with an antibiotic. They should also be treated for dehydration and, if necessary, malnutrition.

 # Care for the child with severe malnutrition

Severely malnourished children have wasting (marasmus) and/or swollen face, hands and feet (kwashiorkor). Treatment is the same for both types of malnutrition.

First prevent or deal with low blood sugar and low body temperature (hypothermia)

- Test blood sugar with a glucose test strip. If low blood sugar is confirmed, give 50 ml of 10% glucose solution **or** sugar water. To make the sugar water, dissolve 5 gm (1 rounded teaspoon) of sugar in 50 ml (3 1/2 tablespoons) of water. If you cannot do the test, assume that all malnourished children have low blood sugar and give them sugar water.

- Check the child's temperature. If it is below 35°C underarm or 35.5°C rectally, start rehydration, if needed and feed the child at once. Put the child on the mother's bare chest and cover them both. If the mother is not there, cover the child, including the head, with a warm blanket. Place a heater or lamp nearby. Do not use hot water bottles.

- Check the child's temperature every two hours until it rises above 36.5°C. Keep the child covered at all times. Feed the child every two hours, using one of the recipes shown on page 93.

Correct the child's electrolyte imbalance

All malnourished children have too much sodium (salt) and too little potassium and magnesium. Their swelling (oedema) is partly a result of this imbalance. Give the child extra potassium and magnesium by feeding the child modified ORS solution, which includes extra potassium and other electrolytes, if it is available. Prepare the child's food without salt, and give foods high in potassium such as carrots and bananas. Mash the food so that it is soft and easy for the child to eat.

Give coconut water if it is available. Coconut water is a very good fluid for patients with diarrhoea and dehydration. It is safe to drink and rich in vitamins and minerals.

Treat any infection

If the child is severely malnourished, the usual signs of infection may be missing. Therefore, all malnourished children should be treated with a broad-spectrum antibiotic, or an antibiotic for a specific infection, such as shigellosis. Also prevent other severe illness by giving measles vaccine to any unimmunized child.

Correct deficiencies in vitamins and minerals

Children with severe malnutrition have vitamin and mineral deficiencies. Give the child a multivitamin supplement to correct these deficiencies and the modified ORS solution if it is available. Give iron only when the child has started to gain weight. If the child has not had vitamin A in the last month, give it now.

Cautiously feed the child

It is important to start feeding the child as soon as possible. Give small, frequent feedings.

The child should have 100 calories per kilogram (kcal) of his or her weight each day and 1-1.5 g protein for each kilogram of weight each day. **If the child is breast-fed, encourage continued breast-feeding.**

If the child is too weak to eat, feed him or her by spoon, dropper or syringe (without the needle), or use a nasogastric tube.

Provide stimulation and loving care

A child who is severely malnourished will be delayed in development. The nurse can help to overcome these delays by providing tender, loving care, and play activities as soon as the child is well enough, and by providing a cheerful, stimulating environment.

Place bright pictures on the wall and point these out to the child. Encourage the parents to bring simple home-made playthings from home and place these within the child's reach.

Talk to the child and tell the child what care you are going to give. Listen to the child and encourage him or her to talk with you.

Encourage the mother to feed and bathe the child and play with him or her. Tell the mother that when the child is back home, she needs to improve his or her development through play, and to feed the child healthy food several times a day.

Children over six months old should be offered food at least five times a day. Tell the mother that good meals need to include cereals and tubers, beans, animal foods such as eggs, milk, fish or meat, small amounts of fat to provide extra calories, and fruit and vegetables.

Care for children with meningitis or malaria

If the child has a fever, look for the source of the infection. The child may have an ear infection, a urinary tract infection, an abscess, etc. If the child has a rash, this could indicate dengue fever, meningococcal disease or measles.

Look for signs of meningitis, such as a stiff neck and irritability. In babies the signs may also include a high-pitched cry, a poor suck and a tense or bulging fontanelle, which is the soft spot on the head. Convulsions may hide the signs of meningitis.

If you see signs of meningitis, prepare to begin intravenous or intramuscular antibiotic treatment. Do not wait for the laboratory results. The sooner you start treatment, the better your chance of success. Carefully watch the child's fluid intake and urine output. Overloading the child with fluids may make brain swelling worse.

In areas where malaria is common, all hospitalized children should have a blood film checked for malaria parasites. As well as malaria, the child may also have severe anaemia, low blood sugar, deep, rapid breathing (acidosis), jaundice, blood coloured urine, or kidney failure. Children with any of these complications are very ill. They should be treated with intramuscular or intravenous quinine and monitored. Check the child for fever and dehydration and for urine output. Watch for signs of anaemia.

Care for the child with acute respiratory infections

The common signs of infection of the respiratory tract are cough, difficult breathing, sore throat, runny nose and ear problems. Fever is also common. All children with a cough or difficulty in breathing should be checked for pneumonia.

Pneumonia

Carefully look at the child's general appearance, effort to breathe and chest movements. Count the child's respiratory

> **Fast breathing is a sign of pneumonia.**

rate for a full minute. Look for breathing movement anywhere on the child's chest or abdomen. If you are not able to see this movement easily, ask the mother to lift the child's shirt. If the child starts to cry or becomes upset, have the mother calm the child again before counting the child's breaths.

If the child is:	Then he or she has fast breathing if you count:
Age 1 week up to 2 months	60 breaths a minute or more
Age 2 months up to 12 months	50 breaths a minute or more
Age 12 months[1] up to 5 years	40 breaths a minute or more

Listen for a harsh noise (stridor), when the child breathes IN.

Listen for wheezing, when the child breathes OUT. Wheezing is caused by a narrowing of the air passages in the lungs.

Check for chest indrawing -- the lower chest wall goes **IN** when the child breathes **IN**.

Based on these signs, classify the child as having:

- no pneumonia

- pneumonia (not severe)

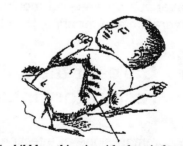

A child breathing in with chest indrawing

---

[1] A child who is exactly 12 months old would have fast breathing if he or she breathed 40 or more times per minute.

- severe pneumonia
- very severe disease.

No pneumonia

A child who does not have chest indrawing and who does not have fast breathing is classified as having no pneumonia.

This child should not be given antibiotics unless he or she has an ear infection.

Give this advice to the mother about home care:

- Keep a young infant warm
- Breast-feed frequently
- Clear the child's nose if it interferes with feeding
- Bring the child back to the clinic quickly if:
    - breathing becomes difficult
    - breathing becomes fast
    - feeding becomes a problem
    - the child or infant becomes sicker
    - the child or infant develops fever.

Pneumonia (not severe)

A child with fast breathing and no chest indrawing is classified as having pneumonia (not severe).

The child should be given antibiotics and home care.

Tell the mother to bring the child to the clinic after two days for reassessment, or earlier if the child gets worse.

Severe pneumonia

If the child has chest indrawing but no cyanosis and can drink, the child is classified as having severe pneumonia.

The child should remain in the hospital and should be given antibiotics. Keep the young infant warm.

(Note: A child with chest indrawing and recurrent wheezing may have asthma rather than severe pneumonia. Children with asthma are managed differently.)

Very severe disease

If the child has any of the following danger signs, he or she has very severe disease:

- cyanosis
- inability to drink
- abnormal sleepiness or difficulty in waking
- stridor in a calm child
- severe malnutrition
- convulsions.

The child may also show chest indrawing.

> *Clinical alert:* In infants under two months of age, suspect severe or very severe disease or other disease with any of the following signs: poor feeding, blue colouring, unusual sleepiness or difficulty in waking, stridor, wheezing, grunting, nasal flaring, fever or low body temperature, or convulsions.

A child who is classified as having very severe disease must have urgent hospital treatment by a qualified doctor.

If the child has cyanosis, or a respiratory rate above 70 breaths per minute, or respiratory distress, give oxygen at a rate of 1-2 litres a minute.

A young infant must be kept warm.

If the child has a high fever, treat the fever with paracetamol.

In areas where there is a lot of malaria, you would usually also give an antimalarial if the child has a fever.

If the child is wheezing, give a bronchodilator such as salbutamol or epinephrine. This will open the air passages and relax bronchospasm. Salbutamol is given by nebulizer and by mouth. Epinephrine is given under the skin (subcutaneous injection).

Encourage the child to drink or breast-feed.

Ear and throat infections

- **If the child has ear pain or pus draining from the ear, he or she may have an ear infection.** Give this child an antibiotic just as you would for pneumonia. Also treat the fever and dry the ear. To do this, roll up a clean, soft cotton cloth. Put it gently in the child's ear, and change it when it is wet. Put in a new dry one and continue until the ear is dry. This is called wicking.

Ear wick

- **If the child has tender swelling behind the ear, there may be a deep infection in the mastoid bone, called mastoiditis.** Treat the child immediately with an antibiotic. He or she may require surgery.

- **If the child has a sore throat with swollen glands in the front of the neck, check the throat**. If the child has a white or yellow pus on the throat, he or she probably has a streptococcal infection. You should treat this child with an antibiotic to prevent rheumatic fever.

Measles, pertussis and diphtheria

Measles, pertussis and diphtheria can be prevented by immunization. Children who have not been immunized can die from acute respiratory infections caused by these diseases. Therefore, they must be treated immediately.

Measles

- A child with measles has fever, a generalized rash and a cough, runny nose and red eyes.

- If a child with measles shows any of the danger signs for pneumonia, or has bloody diarrhoea or an acute ear infection, treat this child with an antibiotic at once. Otherwise do not use antibiotics for measles.

- Children with measles should also receive vitamin A to prevent eye infections. If the child's eyes are clouding and pus is draining from the eyes, he or she should be treated with tetracycline eye ointment as well. Do not use steroidal eye ointments.

- If the child has mouth sores, clean the mouth with clean water and a pinch of salt at least four times a day.

- If the child has diarrhoea, give ORS solution.

- Observe the child closely for danger signs, including inability to drink, decreased consciousness, stridor, or convulsions.

- It is recommended that children with measles be isolated until four days after the start of the rash. Any children in contact with the sick child should receive measles vaccine unless they can prove that they have been immunized.

Pertussis

Pertussis or whooping cough causes violent spasmodic coughing. The child may turn blue or have convulsions or have periods of not breathing (apnea). Pneumonia is the most frequent complication.

Diphtheria

Diphtheria is indicated by a greyish membrane on the throat that cannot be removed by a swab. Children need to be treated immediately with antibiotics and diphtheria antitoxin.

 # Long-lasting illnesses

Some children in hospital are disabled or have chronic illnesses such as heart disease and cancer. These children may have many admissions to hospital. Some children stay in hospital for a very long time.

These children need special care so that they will grow and develop normally. They need to feel loved and safe. They need to feel accepted as individuals, even if they are different. They need to know that their parents are happy and pleased when they learn to do something new. They need to know what they can and what they cannot do. As they grow older, they need to be allowed to decide more things for themselves.

Children also need to learn. They learn by playing, talking and singing.

Give special attention to children in hospital who have long-lasting illnesses and disabilities. Encourage family members to spend as much time with them as possible. Talk with the children. Sing songs with them. Encourage them to tell stories. Try to find things the children can play with. As they get older, involve them in decisions about their daily care. Encourage the family members to find ways to help their children develop normally.

 # Immunizing children

When a child comes into the hospital, always ask the mother if the child has been immunized against tuberculosis, diphtheria, whooping cough, tetanus, poliomyelitis and measles. If the child has not had all these immunizations, give them to the child before he or she is discharged.

If the mother has not been immunized, give her the tetanus vaccine.

 # Involve the family in care

The mother is the child's best caregiver. It is essential to involve her in care.

Listen to the mother to find out how she sees the child's illness. Praise her for bringing the child to the hospital, and show respect for her understanding of the child.

Explain to the mother what you will do for the child and why. Show the mother any equipment you will use, so that she is not frightened by it.

Let the mother hold the child when you give an injection. Tell the mother and the child that it will hurt, so that they are not taken by surprise. Encourage the mother to comfort the child afterwards.

If the child needs ORS solution, show the mother how to feed the child with a spoon and cup.

If the father, grandmother or other family member comes to the hospital or health centre, encourage them to become involved in the child's care.

Teach mothers to care for their children at home

Before the child goes home, give mothers clear instructions about continued care. Make these points clear:

- Make sure the child has plenty of liquids. If the child is breast-feeding, increase breast-feeding.

- Make sure the child does not get too hot or cold.

- Give the child plenty of nutritious food.

- Give medicine correctly.

- Bring the child back if he or she becomes sicker, has difficulty breathing, is breathing fast, or is not able to drink.

- Teach the mother how to monitor the child's health and prevent future problems.

- Tell the mother that the child should have a regular health check up at the local clinic until he or she is school age.

- Show the mother a growth chart. Tell her how to check the child's weight and height to be sure that he or she is growing properly.

- Explain to the mother that the child needs enough to eat to grow properly. Teach her about foods that the child needs. These include:

  - meat, fish, eggs, beans and lentils

- potato, rice, plantain, taro, cassava

- fruits and vegetables

- milk

- some high calorie foods such as oil and sugar.

- Explain the importance of cleanliness, particularly hand-washing. Everyone in the family should wash their hands every morning, before every meal, after going to the toilet, and before helping other family members with eating, dressing, etc.

- Stress the importance of clean foods and clean water. Tell the mother that water from a spring well, pond or river should be boiled. Food should be cooked thoroughly and eaten soon after it is cooked.

- Explain the importance of breast-feeding the baby. Tell her that breast-feeding is much better for the baby than bottle-feeding.

- Explain the importance of having all children immunized against infectious diseases.

- Show the mother how to take care of the child who becomes sick. For example, tell her to give one glass of rehydration fluid every time the child passes a watery or bloody stool. Explain that any fluid, if given early enough, will help to prevent dehydration.

- Tell her that some time-tested home remedies work well such as herbal teas for coughs and colds and coconut water or rice water for diarrhoea. Help her to use these in her care. However, the mother should not rely on home remedies for serious illnesses. She should bring the child to the clinic without delay. Tell the mother to watch for these danger signs:

  - the child is unable to drink or breast-feed

  - the child becomes sicker

- ◆ the child develops a fever
- ◆ the child develops fast breathing or has difficulty breathing
- ◆ the child has blood in the stool
- ◆ the child is lethargic or has convulsions.

- Ask the mother if she has any worries about her own health. Help her get care if she has a health problem. Give her information about how to care for her own health.

Use these basic steps to teach the mother:

- Give information
- Show an example
- Let her practise
- Check her understanding.

Give information

Explain to the mother how to do the task. For example, tell her how to prepare ORS solution or how to soothe a sore throat.

Show an example

Let the mother watch as you mix ORS solution or show her a safe remedy for a sore throat that she could make at home.

Let her practise

Ask the mother to do the task while you watch. For example, have her mix ORS solution or tell you how she will prepare a sore throat remedy at home.

Check her understanding

Do not ask "yes" or "no" questions.

Good questions make the mother tell you why, how or when she will give a treatment. If she cannot answer correctly, give more information or make your instructions clearer.

Always respect the mother.

8 Care for the maternity patient

This chapter is written for the nurse in a small hospital who is working with a doctor or a midwife. Not all small hospitals can provide the special treatments or surgery needed by women who have problems during labour and delivery. Women who are likely to have problems both during pregnancy and at delivery need to be referred to a doctor or midwife who can watch them carefully all through the pregnancy and advise on the right place for delivery. It is the role of the nurse to help decide which women need to be referred to a health facility where they can receive essential obstetrical services. You need to know what signs to look for to see which women to refer.

Check for risk conditions in pregnancy

Look at the antenatal card. Talk to the woman to see if she has any of the following risk conditions:

- Very young or over 35 years of age
- Very short in height
- Less than two years since the birth of the last child
- More than four previous pregnancies
- Previous difficult delivery
- Previous caesarean section

- Baby born dead (stillbirth) or miscarriage in the past

- Premature or very small baby in the past

- Bleeding during a past pregnancy or bleeding now during this pregnancy

- High blood pressure now or during a past pregnancy

- Pregnant with twins now or in the past

- Abdomen larger than normal for the dates of the pregnancy

- Mother has a medical problem, such as severe anaemia, tuberculosis, heart disease, diabetes, malaria, liver disease, kidney disease, urinary tract infection, or a sexually transmitted disease

- Mother malnourished

Women with these risk conditions need to be cared for in a health facility which is staffed and equipped to provide essential obstetrical services, including surgery.

Danger signs during pregnancy

A danger sign means that the woman may have a serious problem. The woman needs immediate care from a midwife or doctor. The most frequent danger signs during pregnancy are:

- Bleeding from the vagina

- Severe headache, dizziness, and blurring of vision

- Puffiness of the face, hands, and feet

- Fever

- Lack of normal colour in the skin (pallor)

- Abdominal pain or tenderness

> **Arrange for immediate medical care if a woman has any danger signs.**

Immediate medical attention may prevent the death of the mother and the child.

 # The three stages of labour

There are three stages of labour:

- The first stage of labour is when the contractions get painful and regular, pushing the baby down and opening up the cervix.

- The second stage of labour is when the cervix is completely open (dilated) and the baby is coming out. The second stage ends when the baby is born.

- The third stage of labour is the time after the baby is born when the placenta separates from the uterus and comes out. The third stage ends when the placenta is out.

 # Decide if the labour is normal or if there are risk signs

When the woman in labour comes to hospital, first decide if she is in normal labour or if she has any risk signs (see below).

Signs of normal labour (first stage of labour)

- Contractions get longer, stronger and closer together.

- The baby starts to come out after 12 hours or less of labour for a woman who has had a baby before; 24 hours or less for the first baby.

- Small amounts of blood-stained mucus "show" may come two to three days before labour starts and continue throughout labour.

- If the bag of water ("the waters") breaks, the colour is clear like ordinary water.

- The mother's temperature stays below 37.8°C.

- The mother's blood pressure remains normal and stays below 140/90.

- The mother's blood pressure does not suddenly drop.

- The mother's pulse is between 60 and 100 beats a minute.

Risk signs in the first stage of labour

If the mother has any of the following risk signs, she will need to deliver her baby at a hospital which can provide essential emergency obstetric services.

- Labour begins before the eighth month of pregnancy.

- The mother has a fever of over 37.8°C.

- The mother's pulse is more than 100 beats a minute.

- The mother has a serious condition called pre-eclampsia. When a mother has pre-eclampsia, her blood pressure may be greater than 140/90 and she may have a swollen face and hands, headaches, and problems with her eyesight.

- The mother has fits (convulsions).

- The bag of waters breaks but labour does not start within eight hours.

- In spite of strong contractions, the labour lasts more than 12 hours for women with previous pregnancies, or 24 hours for the first baby.

- The mother has an unusual amount of bleeding. This includes blood clots, fresh blood or more than "show".

- The mother feels pain between contractions and the womb stays hard.

- The baby's heartbeat is more than 160 beats a minute or less than 110 beats a minute.

- The cord comes out before the baby is born.

If a woman comes to the hospital with any of these signs or if she develops them during labour, she needs emergency obstetric care. She and the baby are in danger of dying. Get help immediately.

How to examine the mother in labour

When the woman arrives at hospital in labour, check the condition of the mother and baby. If there are any risk signs of abnormal labour, arrange for the mother to have expert obstetrical help immediately.

Check the baby's position. Most babies lie with the head down. If the mother is in active labour and the baby's head is up under the ribs or if the baby is lying sidewise, arrange to get the mother to a health facility which has the right emergency obstetrical services. The mother may need surgery to deliver the baby.

Check the baby's heartbeat. A healthy baby's heartbeat is between 120 and 160 beats a minute during labour. It may change and speed up or slow down. It should stay between 120 and 160. Continue to check the baby's heartbeat every half hour during labour.

Check the mother's temperature. Take the mother's temperature when she comes into hospital. Continue to take her temperature at least every four hours while she is in hospital. If you do not have a thermometer, touch her forehead to feel if she is hot. If she feels hot or if she has a temperature above 37.8°C (100°F), she may have an infection. Get medical help and give her plenty of fluids and paracetamol to bring down the fever.

Check the mother's blood pressure. Take the mother's blood pressure when she comes into hospital. Check it every hour. If her blood pressure is going up, check it every 15 to 30 minutes. Remember that if the blood pressure is going up, this is a risk sign. Get medical help.

It is also a risk sign if diastolic blood pressure (the bottom number) suddenly drops 15 or more points. It may mean that she is bleeding inside. Get medical help.

Check the mother's pulse. In early labour, the mother's pulse should be between 60 and 100 beats a minute between contractions. If her pulse is above 100 between contractions, she may have an infection, or be bleeding inside, or be dehydrated.

Ask the mother if her bag of waters has broken. Once the bag of water has broken, germs can move into the womb. To prevent infection to the mother and the baby:

- Do not do vaginal examinations.
- Do not put anything into the mother's vagina.
- Do not let the mother sit in water to bathe.

 # How to prevent problems during the first stage of labour

Good nursing care is important for preventing problems in labour and for monitoring the health of the mother and baby.

The five cleans

Cleanness is the best way to prevent infection.

Clean hands.

Clean perineum.

Clean delivery surface

Cleanness in cutting the umbilical cord.

Cleanness in caring for the newborn baby's cord.

Clinical alert: **Enemas are not necessary and should not be given unless requested by the mother.**

Change the bedding under the mother when it gets wet or soiled. Change cloths and pads when they get very wet. When you change the bedding, check if the mother is bleeding too much, passing blood clots, or passing water which is brown, yellow or green. If you notice any of these risk signs, take action immediately.

Make sure the mother drinks at least one cup of liquid each hour. If the mother is vomiting and cannot drink the cup of liquid at once, have her take small sips after every contraction. Drinks like coconut water, tea with honey or sugar, and fruit juices mixed with water will give her strength for labour. Allow the mother to eat or drink anything she wishes.

Make sure the mother urinates at least once every two hours. If the mother's bladder is very full, it can cause problems in labour and make the labour last much longer.

> *Clinical alert:* **Do not shave the pubic hair.**
> **Shaving can cause infection.**

Make sure the mother changes her position every hour. The mother should not lie flat on her back. This position squeezes the blood vessels and makes blood circulation more difficult.

Check for signs of progress. Signs of progress include:

- contractions get longer, stronger, and closer together

- the mother says contractions feel stronger

- the uterus feels harder during a contraction when you touch it

- the amount of blood-stained mucus (show) increases

- the bag of water breaks

- when the mother has a strong urge to push, the second stage of labour (the birth) is probably near or starting.

> **If the labour lasts longer than 12 hours for women with previous deliveries or 24 hours for the first baby, this is an important risk sign. Get expert medical help for the mother.**

Start making plans to get expert help for the mother when these time limits start getting close.

Help to make the birth safer and easier (second stage of labour)

> **Do not scold or threaten the mother. Upsetting or frightening the mother can slow the birth.**

The midwife or doctor will usually help to deliver the baby. The nurse still has an important role to play.

- Arrange for the mother to give birth in a place that protects her privacy. The room temperature should be at least 25°C so that the baby will not get too cold.

- Make sure that sterile equipment is laid out in a clean place where it will be easy to reach.

- Clean the mother's genitals carefully and gently, using clean or boiled water and a disinfectant if you have it.

- Keep a clean cloth under the mother and very clean cloths close by in case they are needed during the birth. If any stool comes out when the mother is pushing, remove the stool with a clean cloth. If possible, wash the mother again.

- Check the mother's blood pressure every 30 minutes.

- Help the midwife to decide if labour is progressing normally. As long as the baby continues to move down and the mother has strength, there is no need to worry, even if progress is slow. Make sure the mother continues to drink fluid and continues to urinate. If the genitals are not bulging after 30 minutes of strong pushing, this means that the head is not coming down. If the baby is not coming down at all after one hour of pushing, this is a sign that there may be a problem.

Risk signs during birth (the second stage of labour)

> **Clinical alert:** It is dangerous to push on the mother's abdomen to make the baby come out.

- The baby is not born after one to two hours of strong contractions or good pushing.
- Blood gushes out before the baby is born.
- The waters are brown, yellow or green.
- The baby's heartbeat is more than 160 or less than 90 beats a minute.
- The cord is wrapped tightly around the baby's neck.
- The baby gets stuck at the shoulder.
- The baby's feet and legs come out first (breech birth)
- The baby is very small or is more than five weeks earlier than the expected date of delivery.

 # Nursing care in the third stage of labour

Stage 3 begins when the baby is born and ends when the placenta comes out.

Nursing care of the mother

Watch for signs that the placenta has separated from the womb. The placenta usually separates a few minutes after birth, but it may take up to half an hour. Signs that the placenta has separated include:

- a small gush of blood comes from the vagina

- the cord gets longer

- the uterus rises to the navel or above. The top of the uterus (the fundus) may feel rounder and harder.

Once the placenta has separated, the mother should be able to push it out when she has a contraction.

> *Clinical alert:* **Pulling on the cord can be dangerous. Pulling strongly on the cord can break it off from the placenta or can even pull the womb inside out. This can kill the mother.**

Sometimes the midwife will need to pull the placenta out gently by the cord. This is only done after the placenta has separated.

Watch for heavy bleeding. If blood is gushing out or if the woman bleeds more than two cups of blood, this is a danger sign.

Watch for fits (convulsions). If the woman had pre-eclampsia (swelling and high blood pressure) during pregnancy or labour, she may still have fits (convulsions) in the first 24 to 48 hours after giving birth.

After the placenta comes out, the midwife will check the top and bottom of the placenta and the membranes to make sure that everything has come out.

Nursing care of the baby

Dry the baby and keep the baby warm. There is no need to give the baby a bath. The baby will quickly lose body heat if he or she is not dried immediately after birth. Drying also stimulates the baby to breath.

> *Clinical alert:* **There is no need to give a newborn baby a bath.**

After drying, wrap the baby in a dry cloth or put the baby skin-to-skin on the mother's breast or stomach. Then cover the baby. Do not forget to cover the baby's head. You can examine the baby and cut the cord when he or she is lying on the mother. When you care for the baby, keep as much of the body covered as possible.

If the weather is hot, do not wrap the baby in heavy blankets or cloths. Too much heat is dangerous. It will make the baby dehydrated.

Check the baby's health.

- Breathing: A new baby should be trying to breathe within one to two minutes after birth. Normally a newborn baby takes more than 60 breaths a minute in the first two hours after birth.

- Cry: A strong cry means that the baby is breathing well. Do not hit or hurt a baby to make it cry.

- Heartbeat: A new baby's heart should beat between 120 and 160 beats a minute. If the baby's heartbeat is less than 100, get urgent help.

- Movement: A healthy baby should actively move his or her arms and legs.

- Colour: Many babies are blue when they are born, but they quickly become normal colour in one to two minutes. If the baby stays blue, he or she will need help.

Give the baby an intramuscular injection of Vitamin K, if this is the policy in your country. Give the injection in the baby's thigh.

Help the baby to begin breast-feeding. The baby should breast-feed as soon as possible after birth.

Breast milk is all the baby needs for the first four to six months of life. There is no need to give the baby water.

There is no need to give anything else, such as sugared water to the baby, while waiting for the breast milk to come in.

> **Help the mother to breast-feed the baby in the right position.**
>
> The baby's body should be turned towards the mother. The baby's mouth should cover the nipple and the brownish coloured skin (the aereola) around the nipple. The baby's chin should touch the breast.

The first fluid that comes out of the mother's breast after delivery (colostrum) should be given to the baby. Colostrum protects the baby against infection.

Keep the baby with the mother. The baby should be allowed to suck as often as he or she wants, day and night. The more the baby breast-feeds, the more milk will be produced. Both breasts should be used at each feeding.

Breast-feeding should continue even if the baby is sick.

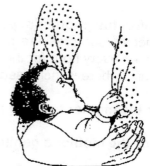

Baby suckling in a good position.

Put medicine in the baby's eyes to prevent blindness. First, gently wipe the baby's eyes clean. Then put 1% tetracycline eye ointment, 0.5% erythromycin ointment or 1% silver nitrate drops in each of the baby's eyes. Do this within the first hour of birth.

 # Nursing care of the mother in the first six hours after the birth

Prevent heavy bleeding. Check the uterus immediately after the placenta comes out. Check it again every 15 minutes for one hour, and then every 30 minutes for the next one to two hours. The top of the uterus (the fundus) should be hard. If it is soft, gently massage the womb until it is hard.

> *Clinical alert:* **If the uterus feels firm but is growing larger, it may be filling up with blood. This is dangerous. Get help urgently.**

Check the mother's pads often. After the birth, it is normal for a woman to bleed as if she is having a normal monthly period. If the mother is bleeding more than this, it can be dangerous. Report it to the doctor or midwife immediately.

Monitor the mother's pulse and blood pressure. Take the mother's blood pressure and pulse every 15 minutes for one hour and then every hour for the next four hours. Report to the doctor or midwife if there is increased pulse or decreased blood pressure.

Help the mother to clean herself, and change her bedding.

Check the mother's genital area for tears and swelling.

Make sure the mother urinates.

Give the mother Vitamin A if this is the policy in your country.

Give liquid to the mother and offer food to her.

 # Nursing care of the baby in the first six hours after birth

Give the family some time alone with the baby. Keep the baby with the mother as much as possible.

Encourage the mother to breast-feed the baby as often as the baby wishes.

Keep the cord stump dry and clean. Cover it with pieces of sterile dry gauze, if available. Do not put anything else on the cord stump.

Give the baby 0.05 cc BCG between the layers of the skin (intradermally) before discharge. In some countries, it is also the policy to immunize the newborn baby against hepatitis B and poliomyelitis.

 # What to do in an emergency while waiting for help

If the baby starts to come out before the midwife or doctor arrives, the nurse will need to deliver the baby.

The baby starts to come out before the midwife arrives. When the baby's head is nearly ready to be born, help the mother to get into a good position. Encourage the mother to push gently. Then when the head is about to come out tell the mother to stop pushing so that the baby's head will come out slowly. Support the baby's head as it comes out.

After the head is born, check if the cord is around the baby's neck. If it is, gently loosen it and slip it over the baby's head and shoulders.

After the baby's head is born, the rest of the body usually slides out easily. Deliver the baby's body. New babies are wet and slippery. Be careful not to drop the baby.

The baby is not breathing or is breathing poorly. If the baby does not cry, suction it out or gently clean the baby's mouth and nose with a clean cloth wrapped around your finger.

If the baby is still not breathing, you will need to revive the baby. Put your mouth over the baby's nose and mouth. Gently blow little puffs of air into the baby at about 30 puffs a minute. Do not blow too hard. Blow little puffs of air from your cheeks, not from your chest. Let the baby breathe out between puffs.

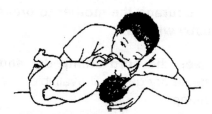

Cover the baby's mouth and nose with your mouth

If the baby dies, tell the mother kindly. Offer to give her the baby to hold. If the other members of the family want to see the baby, let them join the mother. Show that you understand the family's grief. Give them time and privacy to say goodbye to the baby.

The woman is bleeding from the vagina during pregnancy. If the woman has heavy bleeding (a clean pad is soaked in five minutes) and it is not time for her to give birth, get expert medical help for her urgently.

Vaginal bleeding in pregnancy is always a danger sign and heavy bleeding is always an emergency. There are many causes for vaginal bleeding in pregnancy. One of the most frequent causes in first and second trimester of pregnancy is abortion.

When abortions are done by untrained persons, they can be very dangerous. There are many unsafe methods for ending a pregnancy, such as putting something into the vagina or through the cervix, squeezing the womb, or giving modern or plant medicines to start a miscarriage. These and other similar methods can cause severe bleeding, infection, illness, and death. Unsafe abortions are a major cause of death for women.

When a woman comes to hospital complaining of vaginal bleeding, the nurse needs to find out how much she is bleeding, how long she has been bleeding, and the possible cause of the bleeding. Be kind to the woman and do not blame her or scold her if she has had an unsafe abortion. The role of the nurse is to help the woman recover.

All pregnant women who have heavy vaginal bleeding--whatever the cause--will need to be cared for in a health facility that has the staff and equipment necessary to carry out life-saving surgical and medical procedures. If these essential services are not available at your hospital, immediately start intravenous fluids and refer the woman urgently to a referral hospital. If the woman has fever or bad smelling vaginal discharge and abdominal pain, give ampicillin 3 grams orally or procaine penicillin 1.2 million units by intramuscular injection before you transport her or give whatever is the instruction in the local standard procedures manual, if one exists. Give paracetamol 500 mg every four hours if there is fever. Always ask about drug allergies before giving medications.

The woman is bleeding heavily after delivery. If the woman bleeds more than two cups of blood after delivery (500 ml or soaking more than one pad an hour), take quick action to save the mother's life while you are waiting for help.

First, massage the uterus until it gets hard. Then squeeze the uterus between your two hands as hard as you can (bimanual compression), to stop the bleeding.

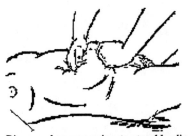

Bimanual compression to stop bleeding

Another very good way to stop bleeding is to press on the aorta (aortic compression). Lie the mother down on a firm surface. Make your hand into a fist. Put your fisted hand one or two fingers below the umbilicus. Press slowly down to the backbone. You will feel the pulse in the aorta. With your other hand, check the femoral pulses in the groin. Keep pressing your fist down until you can no longer feel the femoral pulses. In an emergency, you can teach someone else to compress the aorta so that you can do other things. The compression can be continued for hours, if necessary.

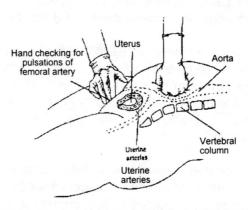

Manual compression of the aorta to stop bleeding

If the bleeding is not greatly reduced within 15 minutes, the mother must get expert medical care urgently. Aortic compression can be continued during transport, if necessary.

Encourage the woman to pass urine. If she has a full bladder and cannot urinate, catheterise her.

Give intravenous fluids if the woman is in shock.

Correct and fast action by the nurse can save the lives of the mother and baby.

9

Caring for the patient who has problems with elimination

The body must have enough fluids to stay healthy. Over half of an adult's weight is made up of fluids. The amount or volume of fluids in the body remains more or less

IN HEALTH

INTAKE = OUTPUT

constant. A person takes in fluid through drinking water and other liquids and through eating foods that contain some liquid. This volume is balanced by the amount of fluid the person loses in breathing, perspiration, urine, and the fluid in solid wastes eliminated from the gastrointestinal tract.

The body fluids contain electrolytes such as sodium, potassium, chloride, phosphate and calcium. In the healthy person these electrolytes are in balance. Some diseases cause fluid or electrolyte imbalances. When a person is ill, the nurse must pay close attention to the amount of fluids the person takes in and excretes, making sure that the fluids and electrolytes are balanced.

There are two types of fluid problems: too little fluid and too much fluid.

Too little fluid

Too little fluid (dehydration) can be the result of taking in too little fluid or losing too much.

Common reasons for taking in too little fluid:

- unable to swallow
- nausea
- lack of appetite
- confusion.

Common reasons for losing too much fluid:

- diarrhoea and vomiting
- excess sweating
- blood loss during surgery
- fluid loss from bad burns
- fever
- too much urination, as with uncontrolled diabetes
- drainage from wounds.

Always look for the signs of dehydration. One of the easiest signs to see is lack of elasticity in the skin tissues. When you pinch normal skin, it immediately goes back to its usual position. If the person is dehydrated, the skin will go back to its flat position more slowly. For adults, the best places to test are the forehead, sternum and inner thigh. Test the abdomen or mid-thigh for children. (Skin elasticity is not always a

If the skin fold does not fall right back to normal, the person is dehydrated

reliable sign in elderly persons, who normally have less skin elasticity.)

Signs of dehydration:

- poor skin elasticity (turgor)
- weight loss
- dry mucous membranes (it is easy to see this in the mouth)
- sunken eyes
- a weak, rapid pulse
- low blood pressure (especially a drop in blood pressure when the person has been lying down and tries to stand up)
- a general feeling of weakness
- thirst
- decreased urine output, darker, more concentrated urine.

 Too much fluid

A sick person may also have too much fluid in his or her body (hypervolemia).

Major causes of fluid overload:

- too much salt (sodium chloride)
- intravenous fluids infused too rapidly
- heart failure, kidney failure, and cirrhosis of the liver
- too much use of steroids.

Signs of too much fluid:

- swelling (oedema), especially in the hands and feet
- puffiness around the eyes
- neck veins which stand out
- weight gain
- fluid build-up in the abdomen (ascites)
- high blood pressure
- a full bounding pulse sound
- slow emptying of the veins in the hand when you lift the hand up
- difficulty with breathing and crackles heard in the lungs when listening with a stethoscope.

 # Electrolyte imbalance

To make sure that the patient does not suffer from fluid or electrolyte imbalances, you must watch and write down the intake of foods and fluids. The fluid output through urine must also be noted. This is especially important for patients who already have imbalances or who are at special risk.

Patients at special risk for electrolyte imbalance:

- the elderly, infants and young children
- patients who cannot take in anything by mouth or whose fluids are restricted
- patients having intravenous fluids
- patients who have had surgery, severe burns or injuries

- patients with urinary catheters or with special drains or suctions

- patients who retain fluids

- patients with congestive heart failure, diabetes, chronic obstructive lung disease or kidney disease

- patients having diuretics.

How to measure and record intake and output

Always measure as exactly as you can the amount of fluids a person takes in and the amount excreted. Many hospitals have what is called an intake-output record or fluid chart. This is where the nurse notes down the fluids the person takes in through intravenous lines (drips), tube feedings and by mouth, and the amount excreted through urine or vomit. If your hospital does not have an intake/output record or fluid chart, make your own.

To monitor intake and output, watch and measure what the patient drinks. It is helpful to make a chart with the measurements of all the kinds of utensils used for fluids in your hospital. For example, the soup bowls used in the hospital may hold 180 ml of fluid. If the patient's family are helping to feed him or her, teach them how to measure what the patient drinks and ask them to write it down or remember it for you.

Intake

Note the amounts of all fluids taken in over a 24-hour period:

- water, milk, juice, tea, cream, soup, coconut water, rice water and other drinks

- foods that become liquid at room temperature such as ice cream, custard and gelatine

- tube feedings

- intravenous fluids

- intravenous medications given with saline solution or otherwise diluted

- any fluids used to irrigate nasogastric tubes or catheters.

You will not be able to measure fluids in the food the patient eats. You can, however, write down what he or she eats or ask the family to remember it for you.

Output

To measure the excretion of fluids over a 24-hour period, make a note of the following:

- urine excreted into a bedpan or urinal or in a catheter drainage bag (or estimated amount if the patient uses the toilet)

- the estimated volume of vomit or watery faeces

- estimated amount of tube drainage

- estimated amount of wound drainage.

If you cannot measure the amount of urine, note the number of times the patient urinated.

If the family helps the patient to the bathroom or helps the patient use a bedpan or urinal, ask them to remember the number of times the patient urinates and whether or not there was anything unusual about the colour. Also ask them to remember and tell you the number of times the patient defecates and whether the stools are watery.

To estimate wound drainage, write down the number of times dressings got wet and needed to be changed.

Add up the amount of intake and output at the end of every shift. Write the numbers on the patient's intake-output sheet or fluid chart.

Compare the amounts with what was recorded previously to see if there have been any changes.

Report too much or too little fluid intake to the nurse in charge or to the doctor.

 ## Help the patient to take in the proper fluids

If patients are taking in too little fluid, try to get them to drink more if possible. Always explain why they need to drink more. Make it easy for them to drink more. As well as water, offer fruit juices, tea, coconut water, etc. Always keep some fluids near the patient. Encourage patients to drink whenever you come into the room. Also, ask any family members present to help patients drink more. People who drink enough should not be thirsty, their mucous membranes will be moist, and their urine should be clear.

> *Clinical alert*: **If the patient is getting fluids intravenously, you must check the flow rate every hour to be sure the patient does not get an overload of fluids or get less than needed.**

Patients who need extra fluids may get them intravenously.

If the patient is overloaded with fluids, explain that he or she will need to limit fluid intake, and why. Use small cups for fluids. This makes the amount seem more than it actually is. Also help the patient to rinse his or her mouth out with water if this can be done without the patient swallowing.

 # Elimination of waste from the body through urination

It is normal to get rid of (eliminate) waste from the body through urination. People can usually feel when their bladder is full. If their muscles are working, they can voluntarily control urination. Many conditions can make people unable to feel fullness, or can cause loss of control over urination.

People with brain or spinal cord injuries, for example, cannot control the emptying of their bladder. Also, elderly people who are confused or demented may not know when their bladder is full. Many elderly people cannot control the muscles used to urinate.

Clinical alert: **Because it is so important to eliminate fluid wastes, you should monitor and note the patient's output of fluids, especially if the patient is at risk for problems. Also, you should encourage the patient to take in enough fluids, since that helps to make sure that waste is eliminated adequately. If the family are helping to provide care, explain to them the importance of getting the patient to drink fluids often.**

Urinary incontinence is being unable to control urine flow.

Urinary retention is being unable to urinate even when the bladder is full.

Other problems with urination include a very frequent need to urinate, unusually large amounts of urine, a need to urinate frequently at night, a need to urinate immediately, and painful urination.

Urination is affected by the amount of fluid the person takes in each day, and by the types of fluids. A person who drinks a great deal of fluid will urinate more than a person who takes in only a little fluid. Alcohol and fluids containing caffeine tend to increase urination. Some medications lead to retention of urine. Others may increase the production of urine. Diabetes also increases urine. Some heart diseases decrease urine production. Diseases of the kidney may lead to a failure of the system for eliminating liquid wastes. This is called renal failure. It is fatal if the body's wastes are not taken away by some other means such as dialysis.

Help the patient to urinate

When patients want to urinate, help them to the toilet if they cannot walk alone. Help them to clean themselves after using the toilet. Help them to wash their hands. Always wash your own hands afterwards. If family members are there, show them how to help with going to the bathroom and making sure that patients are clean after using the toilet. Instruct family members to help patients to wash their hands and then to wash their own hands.

If patients cannot walk to the toilet even with support, help them to use a urinal or bedpan. Give them as much privacy as possible, and clean them afterwards. Then wash your hands.

Urinary catheters

Sometimes patients cannot urinate and you need to put in a catheter.

Catheterization always brings the risk of infection and it should be avoided if at all possible.

Catheterization involves putting a tube called a catheter through the urethra into the bladder. As well as draining urine, catheterization may be used during surgery to keep the bladder empty. There are two kinds of catheters. A straight catheter is used to drain the bladder for a few minutes. A Foley or indwelling catheter stays in place and continues to drain urine.

Always provide privacy for patients when a procedure involves the genital area. Close the door or pull the curtains around the bed.

Before you begin, explain what you are going to do and why. Tell patients that inserting the catheter should not hurt although they may feel some pressure.

Use sterile technique and be extremely careful when putting in a catheter.

If the catheter is not sterile you can bring microorganisms into the bladder and cause infection. If you are not careful in introducing the catheter tube, you can damage the urethra. This is especially likely in the male, whose urethra is longer than in the female.

Taking care of the patient with a catheter

In caring for a patient with an indwelling catheter, the main goal is to prevent infection of the urinary tract.

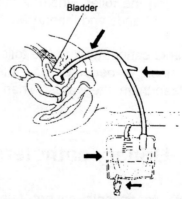

Sites where germs can enter and cause urinary tract infections

The best way to prevent infection is to make sure that the patient drinks a lot of fluid every day, up to three litres. Drinking a lot produces a lot of urine. This keeps the bladder flushed out and stops sediment from sticking in the catheter. Teach the patient and his or her family to check the drainage tube and bag and make sure they are always below the level of the patient's bladder, so that gravity will help the urine flow. Remind the patient never to lie on the tubing and to check it to make sure there are no bends in the tube. Give or help the patient with perineal hygiene twice a day.

Clinical alert: **Never leave the urine bag lying on the floor. The floor is covered with germs which can enter the bag, tubing and urethra. This can cause severe infection or sepsis in the patient.**

Changing the catheter increases the chances of infection. Do not disconnect it unless it is absolutely necessary. Take out the catheter as soon as possible. Infections are easily transmitted by catheters. Always wash your hands carefully before and after catheter care. If sediment gathers in the tubing or drainage bag, or if there is a leak, you need to change the tube and bag. If you change the tubing, you must use strict sterile technique (see the chapter on protecting the patient from infection).

Removing an indwelling catheter

Patients may lose some muscle tone when they have an indwelling catheter. It is helpful to clamp the catheter off for a couple of hours a day for several days before you remove it. This allows the bladder to get fuller, which stimulates the bladder muscles. This helps the patient to regain control of urination after the catheter is removed.

After removal, make sure the patient begins urinating.

Faecal elimination

The body needs to eliminate the solid waste products of digestion (faecal elimination), called passage of stool, or bowel movement. Healthy people may have a bowel movement as often as several times a day or only two or three times a week. People's routines may differ depending on the type of foods they eat and the amount of fluids they take in.

People have two major types of problems with faecal elimination. These problems are constipation and diarrhoea.

Constipation is when small, dry hard stool is passed, or when no stool is passed for a time. Long-lasting constipation can lead to faecal impaction (see the next section).

Diarrhoea is when watery faeces are passed, with frequent defecation. Severe diarrhoea, if untreated, can lead to dehydration and death.

 # How to help the patient who is constipated

Constipation is common in patients who are hospitalized. Lack of movement puts the patient at risk and so do certain drugs. The stress of hospitalization and loss of routines make constipation even more likely.

When you are caring for patients, ask them if they are passing stool, if they are constipated, or if they are passing hard stools.

If patients are constipated, encourage them to take in more fluids. Hot drinks and fruit juices are especially helpful. Also make sure that patients are eating foods containing fibre, such as fresh fruits and vegetables, root crops, peas, beans, lentils, cereals, grains, and wholemeal bread.

Tell patients that they should not ignore the urge to defecate. As soon as they feel the urge, help them to walk to the toilet, or instruct family members to help. If patients cannot walk to the toilet, even with help, provide a bedpan. Always give patients privacy.

Some patients may require a laxative in order to have a bowel movement. If the constipation continues even after a laxative, it may be necessary to give an enema to remove faeces.

Giving an enema

An enema is a solution put into the rectum. It makes the colon bigger, softens the faeces, and lubricates the rectum to make the passage of faeces easier. An enema is also sometimes given to prepare the patient for certain diagnostic tests. Use normal saline solution for the enema. If none is available, you can make a solution by mixing one teaspoon of table salt in 500 ml of water.

Removing an impaction

If none of the above measures are effective, you may occasionally have to take out impacted faeces with your fingers. Put on gloves and lubricate your index finger. Gently insert it into the rectum and loosen and break up the pieces of hard stool. Do this extremely carefully to avoid injuring the mucous membranes of the bowel.

How to help the patient with diarrhoea

In diarrhoea the stools contain more water than normal and are said to be loose or watery. If they contain blood, the diarrhoea is called dysentery. The great dangers of diarrhoea are dehydration and, in the case of children, malnutrition. It is essential to check patients for the clinical signs of dehydration: rapid pulse, low blood pressure, poor skin elasticity, sunken eyes, dry mucous membranes, absence of tears, and weight loss. It is also important to take a stool smear if possible, to look for the cause of the diarrhoea.

Diarrhoea caused by bacteria such as shigella and salmonella, and acute amoebic dysentery and giardiasis, are treated with antibiotics.

Severe cases of cholera are also treated with antibiotics.

Most diarrhoea is caused by viruses. In this case, antibiotic treatment is not recommended.

Even if the patient with diarrhoea does not show signs of dehydration, help the patient to increase fluid intake.

If the patient shows at least two of the signs of dehydration, the condition must be treated at once.

The primary treatment, for both children and adults, is rehydration, by mouth (orally) if possible. If oral rehydration is not possible, then do it through a

> **The primary treatment for diarrhoea is rehydration by mouth**

nasogastric tube or through intravenous fluids. If patients can drink, they are usually given oral rehydration salt solution (ORS) even if they are also being given fluids intravenously.

Patients who are taking antibiotics also need adequate rehydration as well as their medication.

ORS solution comes in already prepared packets to which you add clean water. Make sure that you add the right amount of water.

Always wash your hands before mixing the solution. Use the cleanest water available, preferably boiled water. Cool the water before giving the solution to the patient. Mix a new solution each day in a clean container.

If packages of ORS solution are not available, other fluids which can be used for oral rehydration are coconut water, soups, yoghurt drinks and rice water. Plain clean drinking water should also always be given.

Give the patient one to two cups of fluid every time he or she passes a stool.

How to prevent dehydration in children

Children can get dehydrated very quickly. Teach mothers how to prevent dehydration when the child gets diarrhoea.

The three rules for treating diarrhoea at home are:

1. Give the child more fluids than usual to prevent dehydration

    *   Give ORS solution and other fluids such as soup, rice water, coconut water and plain water.

    *   Give as much of these fluids as the child will take.

    *   Continue giving extra fluids until the diarrhoea stops.

2. Give the child plenty of food to prevent malnutrition.

    *   Continue to breast-feed frequently.

        If the child is not breast-fed, give the usual milk.

    *   If the child is six months or older, or already taking solid food, offer food at least six times a day.

    *   After the diarrhoea stops, give an extra meal each day for two weeks.

3. Take the child to the health worker if the child does not get better in three days or develops any of the following danger signs:

    *   many watery stools
    *   repeated vomiting
    *   strong thirst
    *   eating or drinking poorly
    *   fever
    *   blood in the stool.

It may be necessary to give the fluid to a child with a cup and spoon. Teach the mother how to prepare the ORS and how to give the fluid to her child.

10 Meeting patients' nutritional needs

We need nutrients to maintain the body's functions and to grow. We need water and carbohydrates, proteins, fats, vitamins and minerals. Every cell in the body needs energy. A person must take in enough calories, in the form of carbohydrates, fats, and proteins, to supply that energy. The body also needs the amino acids found in proteins to build and maintain the structure of the cells and larger tissues. Finally, the body needs vitamins and minerals for metabolism and to regulate the many body processes.

To get the right nutrients for the body, a person needs to eat enough foods and a variety of foods. Foods may be divided into groups. Each group contains some of those nutrients.

Breads, cereals, root crops, rice, beans, lentils and sweet potatoes supply complex carbohydrates for energy, some protein, several vitamins and minerals needed to regulate body processes, and fibre, which helps the bowel to work well.

Vegetables and fruits also supply carbohydrates, and they supply many of the vitamins and minerals, particularly vitamins A and C. Fresh fruits and vegetables also contain fibre.

Meat, poultry, fish, eggs and nuts are the major sources of protein for growth and repair of the body's tissues and to fight infections. They also have B vitamins, some minerals, and some fats.

Milk, yoghurt and cheese also supply protein and some fat as well as vitamins and minerals.

Fats, oils and sweets supply mostly fats and carbohydrates and are very high in calories.

The body's need for water is discussed in the chapter on caring for the patient who has problems with elimination. This chapter suggests ways to care for the patient who has trouble eating enough to nourish the body.

 # Nutritional problems of the hospitalized patient

An ill person needs more food than a well one, in order to heal and recover. For example, a patient who has had surgery needs a diet which has a lot of vitamin C and protein since these help with healing. Also, proteins are especially important to fight off infection because the antibodies that the body uses to fight infection are proteins. Often people use up their protein reserves when they have surgery or are injured or have an illness with fever. An adequate diet is essential. Many illnesses, however, make it difficult for a person to eat, or make it hard for the person to digest food.

Conditions making it difficult to get adequate nutrition

- A person with a very sore throat may find it hard to swallow food.

- A person who has a stomach problem may be nauseated by food.

- A person who has a fever is likely to have no appetite.

- Patients who are in the hospital are almost always at risk of getting insufficient nutrients either because of their illness or because of the treatment for their illness.

- Many patients are already undernourished when they enter the hospital.

- The food served in the hospital may be different from the food the patient is accustomed to eating. Patients may not like the hospital food.

- Meals may be served at times when the patients are not accustomed to eating and when they do not feel hungry.

- Patients are often put on a special diet in the hospital to help treat their disease (for example, a person who has had a heart problem will usually be put on a low-salt diet). Patients may not like the change in diet.

- The patient's family may live far away so they cannot bring the foods he or she likes, or the family may not know the right foods to bring, or may not be able to afford the right foods.

 ## How to meet the nutritional needs of the patient

To make sure that the people who are seriously ill or who have just had surgery get enough fluid and at least some calories, they may be fed intravenously until they are able to eat. Intravenous therapy is discussed in the chapter on safe administration of medicines. Intravenous fluids provide enough fluid, but not enough calories. Patients cannot live on intravenous fluids alone. Patients usually go from intravenous feedings to liquids, to a soft diet and then to a regular diet. Sometimes people are able to go straight from liquids to a regular diet.

Liquid diet

Liquids include coffee, soft drinks, fruit juices, coconut water, clear soup or broth and sweetened tea. The person on liquids can also eat gelatine, sugar and hard candies. A liquid diet will give the patient enough fluids and some carbohydrates (from sugar and fruit juices). It will not supply proteins, fats, iron, or enough calories or vitamins. Usually a person should be on a liquid diet for only a short time after surgery or while recovering from acute stomach or intestinal diseases. A patient who has to be on a liquid diet for a long time should be given a nutritional supplement.

Soft diet

A soft diet includes all foods that can be easily chewed and digested. For example, a soft diet might include various cooked, mashed root crops such as taro, kumara, cassava, and yams as well as rice, eggs, very tender lean meat or fish, pasta, tapioca, soft or pureed cooked greens or other vegetables, cooked fruits, bread, and soft desserts. This diet is used for patients who have difficulty chewing and swallowing.

Regular diet

A regular diet is the food the patient normally eats, in particular local foods, which are high in protein, fibre, iron and vitamins.

 Help the patient to eat

Make the patient comfortable. To help a patient who is having trouble eating and who is in pain, it is useful to give pain medication 30 minutes before meal times. This will keep the pain from interfering with eating. For a person who has a fever, give paracetamol or other anti-fever medication before meals to keep the fever from interfering with appetite. Also, avoid doing painful or uncomfortable treatments before meals.

Explain the importance of good nutrition. Explain the importance of eating properly. Encourage the patient to try to eat at least small portions to help with recovery.

Encourage the family to bring foods the patient likes from home. Make sure that the family understands what foods the patient can and cannot eat. Use this opportunity to teach the family about a proper diet. This will help all members of the family as well as the patient. Explain to them the importance of using pasteurized milk, not raw milk, of washing foods such as lettuce which are eaten raw, and of thoroughly cooking meat, poultry and eggs. Tell them to store cooked foods carefully, protect foods from insects and rodents, and keep surfaces clean where food is prepared. Remind them to boil water unless they know it is safe and always wash their hands before preparing food.

Position the patient for eating. If the patient is allowed to sit up, help him or her to do so for meals. It is much easier to eat in this position.

Make the surroundings pleasant. Clean the bed table and make sure there is room for all dishes. Food should be served on a clean tray and should look attractive. Make sure there are eating utensils.

Keep the surrounding area clean and free of unpleasant smells. Remove bedpans, urinals and other such objects from the patient's sight. It is important that the patient's room and table offer a pleasant environment for eating.

Place the food conveniently for the patient. Give help as needed.

Encourage the patient's family to visit at meal times and to help him with eating. Remind them to wash their hands before helping the patient.

If necessary, help the patient eat. Some patients require special help with eating. For example, elderly patients are weak and easily tired. The effort of getting food to their mouth may be more than they can manage. You may need to feed such patients if their families are not there to feed them. Wash your hands first. Ask the patient if he or she would like help. If so, ask what he or she would like to eat first. Feed the patient in small bites. Allow time for chewing and swallowing before offering the next bite. Offer the patient something to drink after every three or four bites. Do not rush the patient or show that you are in a hurry. Use the time to get to know the patient. Take away the eating utensils when the patient has finished and see that they are washed.

11

Care for the patient with limited mobility

Human beings need to be able to move. When people can stand up and move about, they are healthier. Their lungs expand more easily. They are better at digesting food completely. They have good bowel movements, their kidneys function better and their bones and muscles are healthier. When people are ill, they are often unable to move or can move only a little.

Sometimes bed rest or no movement at all is needed to treat a health problem. The rest promotes healing and reduces pain. Long-lasting bed rest or lack of movement can cause serious problems.

Problems caused by prolonged immobility

- Light-headedness

    The blood tends to stay in the legs and feet (called orthostatic hypotension). When the person tries to sit up or stand up, he or she feels light-headed and may faint or fall.

- Infections

    When a patient is lying down and not moving, breathing is more shallow. Pools of fluid can form in the lungs. These pools make it easier for bacteria to grow and can lead to severe infections.

- Weak muscles
- Loss of joint movement (contractures)
- Stiffness and pain in the joints
- Loss of calcium, which makes bones fracture easily
- Constipation (poor bowel movement)
- Poor blood circulation resulting in pressure sores, blood clots or inflammation of the leg veins

The role of the nurse

It is the responsibility of the nurse to:

- help the patient to move as much as possible
- prevent the problems which come from the patient not moving
- help the patient to avoid injury from falling
- help the patient to be able to move independently again, if possible.

 Prevent problems caused by immobility

To prevent light-headedness when the patient stands:

- teach the patient to do leg exercises and other exercises while in bed
- get the patient out of bed as soon as possible
- ask the patient to hang his or her legs over the side of the bed before trying to stand up.

To prevent lung infections:

- teach the patient to do deep breathing and coughing exercises
- change the patient's position every two hours
- make sure that the patient drinks enough fluids.

To prevent loss of joint mobility (contractures) and loss of muscle tone and bone:

- show the patient or a family member how to do range of motion exercises (described below)
- tell the patient to try to increase physical activity gradually.

To prevent constipation:

- make sure the patient takes in enough liquids and other nutrients, especially fruits and vegetables
- help the patient either with a bedpan or, if necessary, a catheter, to get rid of fluid waste and prevent the bladder stretching
- if necessary give the patient a stool softener, or laxative. In extreme cases, give an enema.

To prevent pressure sores:

- change the patient's position every two hours
- keep the bed linen smooth
- keep the patient's skin clean and dry
- make sure that the patient never has one part of the body on top of another part
- if the patient is lying on one side, put a pillow between the legs and flex the upper leg

- use pillows, blankets and towel rolls to support pressure areas

- check good positioning and change of position, with increasing physical activity.

To prevent blood clots (thrombosis) or inflammation of the leg veins (thrombophlebitis):

- do range of motion exercises of the patient's feet and legs

- encourage the patient to get out of bed and walk as soon as possible. Assist the patient if necessary.

 # Correct positioning

Most people change their position constantly and move about even in bed. However, when patients are weak or in pain, or have a fracture, or are paralysed or unconscious, they cannot change position as people normally do. Therefore, they need to be moved or be helped to change position.

Back-lying position

The back-lying position is commonly used to help healing after certain operations.

- The back-lying position is flat on the back, often with a small pillow to support the head.

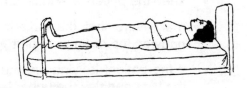

Back-lying position

- The patient's head is in a straight line with his or her back, shoulders, hips and knees. The patient's body should not be twisted.

- The hips move as little as possible, and the patient's toes are pointing up.

- The patient's feet may need to be supported against a firm padded board or a firm pillow to prevent foot drop.

- Arms may be flexed and resting on the stomach, with a pillow under the upper arms.

- A towel roll may be used to separate the legs so that the skin does not rub.

> **Whatever position the patient is in, do not put one part of the body directly on top of another.**

Prone position

The prone position is often used for unconscious patients since it helps with drainage. However, it should be used only for short times with other patients because it makes breathing difficult.

- The prone position is flat on the stomach, again usually with a small pillow under the head and a pillow under the pelvis.

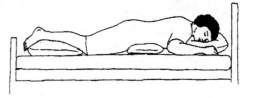

Prone position

- The patient's head is turned to the side.

- The elbows are flexed.

- The toes are off the edge of the mattress, or a roll is placed under the ankles.

Lateral position

The lateral position helps to relieve pressure on the back and the heels for people who are confined to bed or who sit for most of the day. This position is good for resting or sleeping.

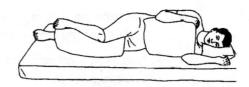

Lateral position

- The patient lies on one side, usually with the top hip and knee bent and supported with a pillow.

- The upper arm is bent, with a pillow under it.

- The patient's feet are supported with a firm pillow, if needed, to prevent foot drop.

Semi-prone position

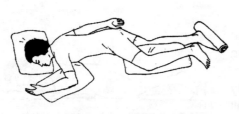

Semi-prone position

The semi-prone position (or Sims' position) is often used for paralysed patients because it reduces pressure on the buttocks and hips. Many people find this position comfortable for sleeping.

- The patient is between a lateral and prone position with one arm behind and one in front. Both legs are flexed.

> ## If a patient cannot change position at all, the nurse should help him or her to change about every two hours.

 ## Moving the patient or changing position

Before trying to move a patient, the nurse should think about the following:

- the patient's own ability to move or help move

- the patient's ability to understand when you explain how to help

- the patient's pain or discomfort in moving.

> **Sometimes, when a patient is in severe pain, it is helpful to give pain relief 30 minutes before the move.**

It is important to think about your own strength and ability to move the patient. In some cases it may take two nurses to move the patient, or even three. If the patient is helpless, always have a second nurse help. Before beginning a move, try to make sure that the sheets are smooth.

Ways to make moving the patient easier

- Stand as close to the bed as possible.

- Lean forward and bend your hips and knees to increase your balance and stability.

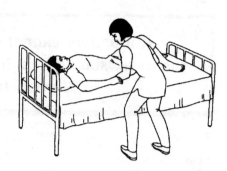

- Face the direction you will be moving the patient in.

- Tighten your buttocks muscles and your stomach muscles to give your body strength to pull or push the patient.

- Stand with your feet apart to get a wide centre of gravity for your own body.

- Rock from your front leg to your back leg to pull, or from your back to your front to push.

- Slide, roll, push or pull the patient instead of lifting, whenever possible.

- Use the long muscles in your arms and legs, not your back muscles, and use your body's weight to help pull or push.

Moving a patient to a wheelchair

Always lock the brakes on both wheels before you move the patient into a wheelchair. Raise the footplates out of the way so that the patient can get into the chair. Put them back once the patient is in the chair.

Exercise the patient

Exercise is essential to keep up muscle strength and joint movement.

People automatically exercise their joints and muscles in normal daily life, when they bathe, comb their hair, dress, eat, write, reach for things, walk, etc. When people are ill and in the hospital, they are not able to exercise as normal. They may need to do range of motion exercises to get them back to their normal level of physical activity.

Range of motion is the term used to describe the complete range of movement of a joint.

Even when patients are able to get up to walk a short distance or sit in a chair, they may need to exercise some joints more.

Range of motion exercises stretch all the muscle groups over each joint.

Active range of motion exercises

The exercises are called active range of motion exercises if patients do the exercise themselves with instruction and possibly some help from the nurse and a family member. The nurse shows patients how to do the exercise to the point of slight resistance. The exercise should not cause pain.

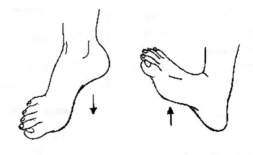

Patient exercising the foot

How to teach the patient and family member to do active range of motion exercises

- Explain what the patient should do.

- Demonstrate the exercise on each joint the patient needs to move.

- Ask the patient to show you in return how he or she will do the exercise. Ask for a return demonstration.

> *Clinical alert:* **Range of motion exercises of the feet and legs are particularly important after surgery, to prevent blood clots from forming in the legs.**

- The patient should do each exercise three times and do the complete set of exercises at least twice a day. If the patient has a weak leg or arm, the other, stronger leg or arm should support the weak one, moving it as far as possible. The nurse or family member can then help the patient to move the limb to the point of resistance.

Passive range of motion exercises

Sometimes a patient is too ill to perform range of motion exercises. In that case the nurse exercises the joints for him or her. These are called passive range of motion exercises.

Some patients begin with passive range of motion exercises and move on to active exercises. Passive range of motion exercises, just like

> *Clinical alert:* **Passive range of motion exercises should not be done on joints that are inflamed.**

active ones, should be done to the point of resistance but not to a point where they cause pain. Each exercise is done by the nurse with the patient three times. The full set of exercises is done at least twice a day.

How to perform passive range of motion exercises

- Explain to the patient what you are going to do and why.

- The patient's feet should be bare, but the body should be covered for privacy.

- Before you begin, tell the patient to say as soon as a movement causes pain, so that you can stop.

- Work on one side of the body first.

- Then move to the other side of the body.

- For each joint that you move, support the patient's limb above and below the joint to avoid muscle strain.

- Move the limb or other body part smoothly and slowly.

- If muscle spasm occurs, stop the movement and press lightly on the muscle until it relaxes.

Exercising the joints

- First exercise the patient's neck joint, while supporting the head and neck.

- Next support the elbow and wrist and move the shoulder through its range of motion.

> **Exercise the joints of patients who cannot move by themselves.**

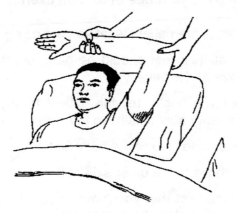

Exercising the shoulder

- Then flex the elbow, the wrist, the fingers and thumb.

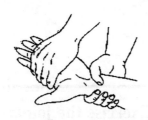 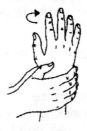 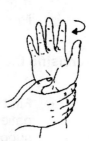

Exercising the wrist

- Supporting the knee and ankle, flex and extend the hip and the knee.

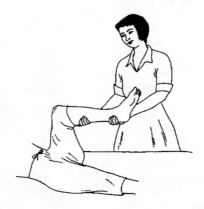

- Move to the ankle and flex it through its full range of motion.

- Next flex the foot and toes.

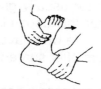

Exercising the foot

- When you have finished, exercise the joints on the patient's other side.

Teach family members to help the patient do range of motion exercises.

 Help the patient to walk

Most people take walking for granted when they are well. After they have been kept in bed, they have difficulty beginning to walk again. Bed rest makes people feel shaky and unsure of their balance. The longer the bed rest, the weaker people feel. Also, those who have had surgery may feel pain when they try to get up and walk.

It is essential to get patients out of bed and walking as soon as possible. The longer people are on bed rest, the more likely they are to suffer complications from lack of movement.

Clinical alert: **Help patients to get up. Help them to walk as soon as possible after surgery or during illness. This speeds up recovery and prevents pneumonia, blood clots and muscle wasting.**

The doctor usually gives an order for getting the patient up. The timing for this depends on the patient's degree of injury or illness. Even people who have had major surgery are often walking within a few hours after surgery.

How to prepare a person for walking

- Check the patient's pulse, respiration and blood pressure, especially if this is the first time up.

- Check the range of motion of the joints the patient will need to use in walking and the muscle strength in his or her legs.

- If the patient is experiencing pain, give pain relief medication 30 minutes before walking, since using the muscles for walking will increase pain.

- Ask the patient to sit up on the side of the bed, and give help if necessary.

The patient should hang his or her legs over the side of the bed for a few minutes and take some deep breaths before standing. Make sure the patient feels no dizziness or light-headedness when standing. Make the patient stand by the side of the bed for a few minutes until he or she feels stable.

> *Clinical alert:* **Check the patient's blood pressure and pulse sitting or standing if there is any dizziness, nausea, or weakness, or if the patient appears pale and sweaty.**

If the patient can walk alone, encourage this but walk close alongside so that you can help if the patient slips or feels faint. You can lock your forearm with the patient's arm and walk together. If the patient seems very unsteady, put one arm around the patient's waist for support and hold onto the arm nearest you, supporting the patient at the elbow. If the patient grows faint and begins to fall, help him or her into the nearest chair. Put the patient's head between his or her knees. When the patient is better, help him or her back to bed. If there is no chair available, help the patient to slide gently down to the floor. Take care that the patient's head does not hit the floor.

Sometimes a patient is very weak and two nurses or a nurse and a family member are needed for support. Each helper should grasp the back of the patient's upper arm with one hand and hold the forearm with the other. If the patient grows faint and starts to fall, grasp the underarms and help him or her to slide to the floor or into a nearby chair.

Use devices to help the patient walk

Many patients must learn to walk with a cane or crutches. Before the patient leaves the hospital, help the patient to decide what he or she will need, help get the equipment and teach the patient how to use it.

Cane

A cane is especially helpful if the patient has one weak leg.

- When the patient is ready to take a step, explain how to move the cane out in front, a little beyond the step, and put it firmly on the floor.

> **Teach the patient to hold the cane on the strong side of his or her body.**

- Next, move the weak leg forward with the patient's weight on the strong leg and the cane.
- Once the weak leg is on the floor, move the strong leg forward. The patient's weight is supported by the cane and the weak leg.
- Repeat the process.

Crutches

Crutches may be temporary or, for some people permanent. The most common type of crutch fits under the arm and has a bar for the hand.

The crutches must be the right height for the patient and the arm bar must be right.

When walking with crutches, the patient's weight needs to be supported by the shoulders and arms, not the underarms. The elbows should be bent.

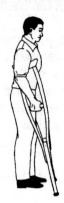

 # Care for the person in a cast

Patients with broken bones, severe sprains, or dislocated joints are often put in a cast. This stops the bone and tissue moving until they heal. If the cast is on the foot or leg, the toes are usually left open. If it is on the hand or arm, the fingers are left open. To prevent swelling (oedema), the person in a cast should keep the casted area raised above the level of the heart, as much as possible.

The nurse needs to watch the patient carefully for signs of problems.

- If the cast is on the foot or leg, check the colour, temperature, size, movement and feeling of the toes. Compare these results with the other foot.

- If the cast is on the hand or arm, check the fingers and compare them with the other hand.

- Check capillary refill. A pink colour should return quickly to a nail bed when you press on it.

- Look at the skin around the edges of the cast for signs of irritation. If the cast has a rough, irritating edge, cover it with adhesive tape, and tell the doctor. Do not cut the cast.

Clinical alert: **If the skin is pale, bluish, or cold, there is a problem with circulation. Tell the doctor immediately.**

- Look at the skin colour of the fingers or toes, or other area affected by the cast.

- If the fingers or toes or other area affected by the cast are swollen, that also indicates a problem with circulation. Raise the casted area higher and tell the doctor.

- Check the temperature of the area around the cast. If the area is warmer than the surrounding skin, that is a sign of infection. If the area is colder than the surrounding skin, that is a sign of a problem with circulation. The nurse should call the doctor if the area around the cast is warmer or colder than the normal.

- Smell the cast. A bad smell coming from the cast indicates infection.

- Ask the patient about pain. If there is increased pain or burning under the cast, that may also be a sign of infection, or it may be a sign that the cast is too tight.

Areas where pressure sores can develop in a long leg cast

> *Clinical alert:* **If a patient complains of increasing pain or severe pain in a casted arm or leg, tell the doctor immediately. Swelling under the cast could be interfering with blood flow and nerve function in the limb.**

- Check the colour, temperature, size and sensation of the area affected by the cast hourly for the first 8-12 hours after surgery or after cast application; then check at least once every day.

Advising the patient and family about care of the cast

Show the patient and family members how to prevent problems and watch for signs of complications. Give these instructions:

- Keep the casted area raised.

- Do not put anything down the cast to scratch an itching area.

- Do not get the cast wet.

- Check the colour, temperature, size and feeling of the casted area.

- Tell the nurse if the patient feels any numbness or tingling of the casted area, if the patient feels increased pain, or if the patient has any chest pain or shortness of breath.

Tell the patient and family members to exercise the patient's other joints while in bed. If the cast is on the foot or leg, the nurse or family members will need to help the patient walk on crutches. The patient should eat a balanced diet and drink extra water to prevent constipation because of the reduced movement.

12 Care for the surgical patient

Many of the people in hospital are there for surgery. People need surgery for many reasons: to find the reason for a problem, to help reduce that problem, or to mend, replace or take out tissue or organs. Surgery may also be carried out as an emergency, to save the patient's life.

Preparing the patient for surgery

Before surgery, the doctor asks for tests and examinations of the patient. These give information on the problem requiring surgery. They also tell the doctor about the patient's health and the risks of surgery. The nurse plays a major role in getting the patient ready for the operation.

- The nurse checks the patient's health.
- The nurse makes sure that all investigations are carried out.
- The nurse explains to the patient what will happen before surgery and what he or she will feel after the surgery.
- The nurse physically prepares the patient for the operation.
- The nurse shows the patient what to do to help with recovery after surgery.

Surgery disrupts a patient's life. It brings anxiety and fear, pain and discomfort. By giving the patient information and reassurance, you can calm those fears and prepare his or her mind for the experience. A well prepared patient will find the experience of surgery much easier.

- If the patient goes into hospital before the operation, explain as soon as the patient arrives what tests will be done and why they must be done.

- The day before the surgery, explain to the patient how to prepare. For example, a patient may have an enema before bowel surgery.

- Explain that the patient must not eat or drink for 8-12 hours before the surgery. This is because under anaesthesia the patient might vomit and choke.

- Ask the patient to bathe in the morning, remove all jewellery, makeup, eyeglasses, dentures, etc., before going to the operating room.

- If the patient has family members there, tell them where they will be able to wait during the operation.

- Explain to the patient how the operating theatre and recovery room are set up. Tell him or her that staff members will be wearing surgical scrubs and masks. Tell the patient that after the surgery, he or she will go to the recovery room for close monitoring. The patient may have an oxygen mask, a blood pressure cuff on his or her arm and other monitoring equipment attached.

- Teach the patient to do coughing and deep breathing exercises. These will be needed after the surgery to speed up recovery and prevent complications.

◆ First, show the patient how to breath deeply. Inhale slowly through the nose while feeling the diaphragm move out and up. Hold your breath for a second or two, then exhale through the nose or through the mouth with a whooshing sound.

◆ Then ask the patient to sit up and show you how he or she can do the deep breathing. After this, ask the patient to breathe in deeply and then cough.

◆ Next show the patient how to support the stomach area by holding a pillow firmly against it while coughing. This will protect the surgical incision and reduce pain when coughing.

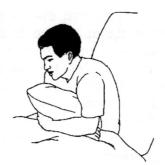

◆ Show the patient how to turn in bed, holding a small pillow against the incision to support it.

Supporting the stomach area with a pillow while coughing

Tell the patient to begin these coughing and deep breathing exercises as soon as possible after surgery. They should be done at least four times a day, taking five breaths and coughing twice each time.

• Show the patient these leg exercises to do after surgery.

◆ Pull the knees up, then straighten the legs and press the back of the knees down.

- ◆ Pull one knee up at a time, then extend that leg outwards.

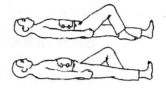

- ◆ Next hold the legs straight and move the feet in circles.

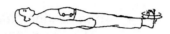

Exercising legs and feet after surgery

- ◆ Raise one leg while holding the other knee flexed.

Make sure that the patient understands that he or she will have pain relief after surgery. Tell the patient that it is safe to take narcotic pain medications after surgery. Explain that they will heal better if they are free from pain. Remind the patient to tell the hospital staff if he or she is in pain.

> **Tell the patient why it is important to walk as soon as possible after surgery.**

 # Immediately before surgery

Patients should empty their bladder before surgery. They should take out false teeth, hairpins and clips, and take off glasses, rings, nail polish, lipstick, etc.

The patient may be given a narcotic before the surgery and atropine to dry the secretions of the mouth. Sometimes a tranquillizer is also given. Often, however, no medications are ordered until the patient is taken to the operating theatre.

Wash the skin around the site of the incision and clean it with an antimicrobial agent. The clean area must be larger than the incision so that if the cut needs to be made bigger, the skin is properly prepared. The area should not routinely be shaved because that can make the skin vulnerable to infection. If there is a lot of hair and it absolutely must be removed, it is better to clip the hair. Only shave if it is essential.

Usually an intravenous line with saline solution is started before surgery. This may be done in the patient's room, or in the operating theatre. If there is a high risk of infection, usually antibiotics are given intravenously.

Prepare the family for the surgery. After the patient is taken to the operating theatre, tell the family how long the surgery is likely to take. Show them where they can wait comfortably. Promise to give them information as soon as you can. It is very helpful for a nurse to come out of the operating theatre from time to time to tell the family that the surgery is progressing well. If there are serious problems, however, it is not useful to inform the family until you have a clear idea of what is going to happen. As soon as the surgery is finished and the patient has been moved to the recovery room or to a hospital room, tell the family. Tell them when they will be able to see the patient. Let them visit as soon as the patient is in a stable condition.

 # The nurse's role during and immediately after surgery

- Before the surgery begins, operating theatre nurses check how the patient is (vital signs, etc.), get the patient ready for the surgery, and help to prepare the sterile field for the surgery.

- During the operation, nurses open supplies and pass them out, manage any tubes or drains, and look after intravenous medications and solutions. The nurses make sure that the patient is safe during surgery, that there is surgical asepsis and a sterile field, and that the surgical positioning does not hurt the patient. The nurse counts needles and gauze swabs used during the operation to make sure that nothing is left inside the patient after surgery.

- In many countries, nurses have been taught to give the anaesthesia. In other countries, this is the role of the doctor.

- After the surgery, the patient usually goes to a recovery room or intensive care unit where nurses check how the patient is and take care of him or her. In the recovery room, the patient is usually put onto his or her side, with no head pillow. This position keeps the airway open and allows drainage of any mucus or vomit. Patients who have had a spinal anaesthetic must lie flat. The patient's upper arm has a pillow under it, so that it does not stop the chest moving out to breathe. The patient is kept warm with blankets. All monitoring equipment, IVs, drains, and catheters are secured.

- Nurses keep a careful watch on the patient's airway, breathing rate and depth, and the colour of the mucous membranes and nail beds. The patient's level of alertness, pulse, blood pressure and temperature are carefully monitored and recorded. Usually the patient is still using the artificial airway. The nurse needs to suction the pharynx until the coughing reflex returns.

- Patients wake up from the anaesthesia and get back their reflexes at different speeds. To help them wake up, the nurse can call their name and repeatedly tell them that the surgery is finished. A parent should be at the bedside to comfort a child when he or she wakes up. As the vital signs stabilize and they begin to awaken, the nurse asks patients to take several deep breaths every five to ten minutes. Patients' position is changed every 10 to 15 minutes.

 # Care for the patient after surgery

Patients are usually taken to a regular ward or unit, once they are awake, with their reflexes working, and their breathing, pulse, blood pressure and temperature stable. In cases of high risk or very complicated surgery, patients may remain in an intensive care unit to have special nursing care.

Once back from surgery, the nurse looks at the doctor's orders and checks how the patient is.

- **First look at the patient's airway and breathing. Check the colour of the lips and nail beds**. Check the skin colour and temperature. The skin, including mucous membranes, lips and nail beds, should be pink. If it is bluish or the skin is cool and moist, the patient may be having problems with breathing, blood pressure or circulation.

- **Check the patient's level of consciousness**. The patient should be fully awake though he or she will probably feel sleepy.

- **Take the patient's vital signs**. If they are not fully stable, take them every 15 minutes until they are stable. If the patient has a weak, rapid pulse, low blood pressure, pale, clammy skin and rapid breathing, there may be internal bleeding. If you suspect that there is too much bleeding or internal bleeding, make sure that the patient has an intravenous drip and oxygen. Immediately notify the nurse in charge or the doctor. Once the vital signs are stable, take them every hour for the first day after the operation.

- **Check the patient's bandages and the sheets under the patient.** If there is a lot of blood on the bandages or bedclothes under the patient, he or she may be haemorrhaging. You should call the nurse in charge immediately. If for any reason you feel that the patient is not completely stable or you are concerned about the breathing, vital signs or possible blood loss, make sure that the patient is monitored continuously. Do not hesitate to ask the nurse in charge or the doctor to check the patient.

- **Carefully watch the amount of fluid the patient takes in and the fluid output**. Most patients will continue to be given fluids intravenously for a period after surgery. This makes sure that the fluids lost during surgery are replaced. At the same time, however, take care that the patient does not take in more fluid than the body can handle. Look again at the doctor's order for the amount of fluid for the patient. Check the IV flow rate to make sure that the patient is getting the right amount of fluid.

  Many patients are thirsty when they wake up from anaesthesia. Give them a wet cloth to wet their mouth until they are allowed to have water by mouth. Then when the patients are allowed to drink, give them small amounts of water until you are sure that they will not vomit.

- **Recheck the flow rate and operation of the IV line every hour.** Also check the level of IV fluid in the bag or bottle, to make sure that the patient has had the right amount of fluid each hour. Check any drainage tubes to be sure they are working properly.

- **Write all your initial and ongoing assessments on the patient's chart**, including the patient's vital signs, consciousness, skin colour, bloody drainage, and fluid intake.

How to help the surgical patient to recover

Control post-operative pain

Check the patient's pain level and location. Give the patient the pain relief ordered by the doctor, regularly and on schedule.

Pain is extremely uncomfortable for the patient. It also slows recovery and can lead to complications. There is usually most pain for the first few days after surgery. After that it begins to subside slowly. On the first day after surgery, pain medicine is usually given every three to four hours. The medication is often given intravenously. By the second or third day the patient may be able to take pain medication by mouth.

If the patient refuses the medicine because there is no pain, tell him or her that pain control works best if the medication is given before the pain becomes intense.

The instruction PRN allows the nurse to judge when to give medicine. Patients sometimes do not get all the medicine for pain they need. Make sure the patient gets enough pain medication.

> **Always give pain medication before getting the patient up to walk and before bedtime.**

Make sure that the patient is warm and comfortable. Pain increases with tension. Help the patient to relax with back rubs and other comfort measures.

Make sure fluid intake is adequate

It is important that patients have enough fluids. Check patients for signs of dehydration or fluid overload. These signs are: dry mucous membranes, poor skin elasticity (turgor), thirst and small amounts of concentrated urine. Signs of fluid overload are: difficulty in breathing, distended neck veins, sounds or crackles in the lungs and swelling (oedema).

The patient may be on intravenous fluids for a couple of days after surgery. This depends on how serious the surgery was. Before moving the patient on to taking liquids by mouth, check the bowel sounds by listening through a stethoscope on the patient's abdomen. Gurgling sounds in the intestines are a sign of peristalsis. Listen once or twice daily until you hear bowel sounds. After the intravenous fluids stop, give small sips of water to start with. Then move on to other fluids. Make sure the patient gets enough fluids. This prevents dehydration, keeps mucus from becoming thick and helps to prevent constipation.

Check urinary output

It is essential that the patient urinates. The patient may still have a urinary catheter for a time after surgery. If not, you must help the patient to urinate. Low intake of fluids and continued catheterization can lead to urinary infections. Retention of urine can lead to kidney problems.

If the patient does not urinate within eight hours of surgery, inform the doctor.

Carefully record the amount of fluid taken in and the amount urinated. If the patient is getting enough fluid by mouth or intravenously, the urine should be clear.

Turn and exercise the patient

Patients need to be turned from side to side every two hours. They should get up to walk as soon as possible after the surgery. Usually patients begin walking on the evening of the first day of surgery. Make sure patients are comfortable and their pain is controlled. Ask them to sit on the side of the bed for a while, with the feet hanging down. Then help them to walk. If a patient appears pale or has clammy skin and dizziness when he or she stands up or walks, check the blood pressure and pulse to make sure they are normal.

Good circulation to the feet and legs is important after surgery. A thrombus or clot in a leg vein can come loose and become an embolus that moves to the lungs or heart and obstructs an artery. Leg clots are extremely dangerous. Leg exercises, early walking, plenty of fluids and elastic stockings, if available, are the best way to prevent clots in the veins.

Watch the patient's skin for signs of inflammation, which are usually associated with a clot. Look for a swollen, red area that is warm to the touch and painful, a vein that feels hard, and aching or cramping. There may be a clot if the patient feels discomfort when the foot is flexed.

To prevent clots, encourage the patient to do leg and foot exercises every hour or every two hours whenever he or she is awake.

Encourage coughing and deep breathing

The patient should do coughing and deep breathing exercises every two hours for the first day or so after surgery. The exercises are continued until the patient is up and walking regularly. If the patient learns these exercises before surgery, they will seem easier. Help the patient to support the incision if he or she is in pain. If the patient cannot cough up anything, he or she may need suctioning.

Provide an adequate diet

The patient will move from fluids to a soft diet and then a regular diet. Good fluid intake and early walking help to prevent urinary tract infections, constipation or abdominal distension, and gas left in the intestines. The patient must eat enough healthy food to get the proteins, calories and vitamins to heal the surgical wound and his body.

Check bowel function

Check that the patient is able to get rid of bowel wastes and that the stools are soft. The signs of constipation are: abdominal swelling, pain and no stool or hard stools.

 ## Watching the patient for complications

Watch carefully for the signs of complications after surgery.

- **Pneumonia and collapse of the small air sacs (alveoli) in the lung (called atelectasis)**. The signs of pneumonia or atelectasis include: fever, shortness of breath or fast breathing, chest pain, cough, bloody or infected sputum, and decreased breath sounds or crackling sounds (crepitations) heard in the lung with a stethoscope. Sometimes patients also have bluish coloured mucous membranes and nail beds.

Sudden chest pain and shortness of breath, blue colour, apprehension and the signs of shock (low blood pressure and a very rapid pulse) indicate a blood clot or air embolis in one of the blood vessels in the lung (pulmonary embolism).

- **Haemorrhage**

The signs of haemorrhage may include bloody bandages and bedclothes. If the patient is bleeding internally, you may nct see those signs. One of the first signs of blood loss is increased breathing. Later signs include a rapid weak pulse, low blood pressure, cold, clammy, pale skin, and reduced amount of urine.

- **Urinary problems**

The signs of urinary retention are: the inability to urinate or urinating in small amounts, a stretched bladder, and discomfort in the bladder region. Signs of a urinary tract infection include burning when urinating, a sense of urgency, pain in the lower abdomen, cloudy urine and sometimes a fever.

- **Wound infections**

Caring for the patient's wound and helping it heal are major responsibilities of the nurse. If healing is delayed, the wound is more likely to become infected.

Signs of infection include redness, tenderness, infected discharge, a bad smell in the wound, and fever. The patient may also have a faster pulse rate and faster breathing.

To prevent infection, always wash your hands before caring for the patient's wound. Use sterile technique and sterile dressings if possible.

Do your best to keep the wound area as clean as possible. Change the dressings over wounds when the dressings become wet.

When you change the dressing, clean the wound with sterile saline solution.

Use sterile technique and sterile instruments to remove sutures. Look carefully at the sutures you have removed to make sure all suture material has come out. Suture material left in the wound can cause an infection.

You can use bandages to support or immobilize a wound, secure a dressing or put pressure on an area of the body. When possible, bandage the body part in its normal position. Leave the end of the body part (for example, a toe) exposed so that you can check blood circulation.

Discharging the patient

The health team aims to make the hospital stay as short as possible, and the return home as easy as possible. Before discharge, give the patient and family information about activities and exercise, hygiene, wound care, any medications and follow-up appointments. Encourage the patient to ask questions.

This is discussed further in the chapter on preparing the patient for discharge.

13

Care for the patient in pain

Pain is the most common reason for seeking medical care. Many of the patients the nurse sees are in pain. Their pain causes suffering and interferes with healing. It is the nurse's responsibility to do everything possible to ease the patient's pain. The nurse can never know whether another person is experiencing pain or not, or how much pain that person is feeling. Pain is a personal feeling that cannot be accurately described or measured. The nurse cannot feel the patient's pain or see it. The nurse has to believe in that pain and trust the person's judgement of how severe the pain is.

Assess the patient's pain

To work out how to manage a patient's pain, the nurse must first know where it is (location), what sort of pain it is (quality), and how strong it is (intensity). For surgery patients, burn patients, and patients who have experienced trauma, that information is usually obvious. For other patients, the nurse may need to ask about these details. It may also be useful to ask about what brings on the pain or makes it worse, things that seem to relieve the pain, other symptoms that go with the pain and the effects of the pain.

Here are questions to ask a patient who appears to be in severe acute pain:

- Where is your pain?

- Will you describe the pain for me? What does it feel like?

- How severe is your pain?

These questions will provide the basic information needed to provide relief for the pain. In addition, ask the patient if he or she is taking any other medications. Ask if the patient is allergic to any pain medications.

If it is not clear whether the patient is in pain, begin by simply asking:

- Are you in pain?

Here are other questions that you might ask, especially about chronic or recurring pain, or pain that is difficult to identify:

- When did the pain start? How long have you had it?

- Are you in pain all the time? If not, how long does the pain usually last?

- What usually makes the pain come? What makes it worse?

- What seems to help the pain to go?

- Do you have other symptoms just before or during or after your pain (for example, nausea, blurred vision, dizziness, and shortness of breath)?

- Does the pain affect your sleeping, eating, working, and other activities?

- What do you usually do to try to help the pain to go?

Location of pain

Pain may be felt in one place and be easy to identify. It may be felt in many areas of the body, especially if it is coming from internal organs. Sometimes pain may go out from the place of internal injury to other body parts. Occasionally pain is caused in one place and felt in another (referred pain). Some patients feel what is called phantom pain. This is pain in a body part that has already been cut off. It can continue long after the cut has healed. To help the patient to say where the pain is, you can use a chart of the body or a picture of a person. Ask the patient to point to the place where it hurts. This is especially helpful with children.

Character of pain

Sometimes giving people a list of adjectives may help them to describe their pain. Words commonly used for pain include: sharp, throbbing, burning, searing, stinging, intense, shooting, dull, steady, aching, radiating, pricking, pressing, rubbing, etc. If the patient has these words to choose from, he or she can pick out the ones that apply.

How to identify the patient in pain

Sometimes you can get an idea of the patient's pain simply by looking at him or her. People in pain often clench their teeth, shut their eyes tightly, bite the lower lip and grimace. They may have a beaten look and dull eyes. A person in pain often holds that part of the body still. The person may rub the sore body part. Body movements such as tossing and turning in bed can also indicate pain. People in pain may also moan or cry out. They may be sweating, appear pale or have rapid or shallow breathing.

Patients may suffer more or less from pain, depending on what it means to them. For example, a woman in childbirth may find it easy to stand her pain. She knows that she will have a baby. A person with chronic back pain who is miserable and cannot make the pain stop may not find it easy to stand. Some patients learn ways to cope with pain that make it more tolerable for them. Others do not seem able to cope with pain.

> **Patients respond differently to pain**

A patient's response to pain may also be affected by background and culture. One person may say the pain is not so serious when the family is there, while another tries to get sympathy from family members. One person may say nothing about the pain while another cries out or complains. One patient may want quick relief while another may think pain relief is a sign of weakness or think that pain medication is addictive.

 # How to manage the patient's pain

Here are the keys to effective pain management:

- **Show that you recognize the patient's pain and respond with a caring attitude**.

- **Listen carefully to what the patient says about the pain.**

- **Act to relieve the pain**. In cases of acute pain such as surgery or trauma, it is especially important to act quickly to relieve the pain. Pain can lead to complications and delay recovery. (Do not, however, give pain medication to a patient with acute pain in the abdomen until the problem has been found.)

- **Give pain relief before the pain becomes severe**. If the patient's pain continues, you must give medication on a regular schedule instead of waiting until the patient asks for help. Scheduled doses maintain consistent blood levels and prevent severe pain. This means that less medicine is needed to control the pain. If variable drug dosages have been prescribed (for example, intramuscular morphine 5 to 15 mg every three to four hours), ask the patient about the pain and adjust the dosage to make sure that the patient's pain is controlled.

Pain medication

Drug management involves the use of narcotic opiates, and non-steroidal anti-inflammatory drugs and other analgesics.

Narcotic analgesics

Narcotics relieve pain and give a sense of euphoria. Narcotics like morphine provide maximum pain relief. The dose can be steadily increased to relieve pain. Morphine is the best drug for very severe pain and for the terminally ill, whose pain may steadily increase.

Pethidine is also an effective narcotic analgesic which can be used as an alternative to morphine. But it is not as long-lasting as morphine and is not as effective as morphine for patients who are dying in severe pain. Codeine is a narcotic which can be given by mouth for moderate pain.

Paracetamol or other anti-inflammatory drugs and narcotics work well together. They provide better pain relief than either drug given alone. An effective dose of paracetamol or aspirin for pain relief is between 650 and 1000 mg. Doses of narcotics vary, and you must know the ranges of effective doses. Doses vary depending on how the drug is given.

Administration of narcotics

Narcotics can be given in several different ways. They are given most commonly by oral, intramuscular, or intravenous routes as an intravenous bolus or a continuous intravenous infusion. Oral administration is the easiest route. However, the effect of most opiate narcotics only lasts about four hours. This means that patients taking morphine or other opiates by mouth have to be woken up in the night to control their pain properly. There are some long acting forms of morphine, with a duration of eight hours. There is also a new liquid morphine for those who cannot swallow pills.

Several narcotic opiates are available as suppositories. This route of administration is particularly helpful for patients who cannot swallow or who have nausea and vomiting.

Patients whose pain cannot be controlled by oral medication have their medication injected under the skin (subcutaneous injection). Pain relief can also be given into the muscle. This is not desirable because it is painful, the drugs absorption varies and the shot must be repeated every three to four hours. Giving drugs intravenously is rapid and effective. It is useful for patients in acute pain. Some large hospitals now have patient-controlled pain relief. Pumps give the opiate when the patient pushes a button.

Patient-controlled pain relief is also possible by giving the patient a supply of liquid morphine.

The use of narcotic analgesics is normally controlled by various regulations and procedures to prevent misuse and to comply with international conventions on narcotic drugs. Access to narcotic drugs may be difficult because these drugs are normally kept under locked storage. Health workers are required to keep detailed records of the use of these drugs. This sometimes discourages the use of narcotic analgesics because it adds to the workload and responsibility of the doctors and nurses. But the well-being of the patient must be the main consideration of the nurse. Do not let this extra work stop you from using these effective analgesics.

Side effects of narcotic analgesics

Narcotics all have side effects. You must review these side effects when giving any narcotic.

Respiratory depression: Narcotics may make the patient breathe less. This respiratory depression is the most dangerous side effect. Also, all narcotics make the patient sleepy to begin with.

Check the patient's alertness and breathing before giving any narcotic. This information will help you to decide whether the patient is having breathing

> *Clinical alert:* **If the patient's breathing is reduced, give a drug to reverse the effects of the narcotic, such as naloxone hydrochloride (Narcan) until breathing returns to normal.**

problems or is too sedated. If you see either of these problems, the dose is too large and you should obtain an order from the doctor to reduce the dose immediately.

The amount of sedation from narcotic analgesics will go down gradually on its own after the patient has taken the drug for three to five days.

As well as reducing breathing, narcotic analgesics have other side effects. These include constipation, itching (pruritus) and rarely, inability to urinate (urinary retention).

For **constipation**, increase the patient's fluid intake, increase fibre and bulk-forming agents in the diet, increase exercise and if necessary, use stool softeners or a laxative. Nausea and vomiting will gradually stop. Give an antiemetic until they stop. The patient may prefer to change the analgesic.

For **pruritus** (itching), use cool packs and lotions and give the patient an antihistamine. The most common antihistamine is promethazine (phenergan). Always have this available whenever drugs are given, to counteract reactions.

If the patient suffers **urinary retention** (inability to urinate), the nurse may need to catheterise the patient, or administer a narcotic antagonist drug such as Narcan.

Non-narcotic analgesics

Non-narcotics or non-steroidal anti-inflammatory drugs include aspirin, acetaminophen and ibuprofen. They can work as pain relief and also bring down fever. Their most common side-effect is indigestion, or in extreme cases stomach ulcers and gastric bleeding. This can be prevented by eating some food when taking the medication.

Adjuvant analgesics are drugs which were not developed for pain relief but which can reduce some types of pain, especially chronic pain. These drugs include mild sedatives or tranquillisers. They can reduce muscle spasms as well as anxiety and tension, which may increase pain. Antidepressants such as amitriptyline hydrochloride may also help with pain. Anticonvulsants such as carbamazepine can control the pain of herpes zoster (shingles) and diabetic nerve problems, such as pain in the feet.

You should check patients frequently who may be in acute pain, such as patients after surgery. Check every two hours for the first 24 hours after surgery and then every three to four hours until discharge. Give narcotic analgesics and non-steroidal anti-inflammatory drugs (NSAIDs) as the doctor orders. The NSAIDs increase the pain relief provided by narcotics. Pain is less severe if relief medication is given on a schedule. Do not wait until patients are in such pain that they ask for relief.

When patients are not clear about the cause of pain and the amount of pain, it is helpful to follow the three-step ladder approach suggested by the World Health Organization for cancer pain. This approach is equally useful for pain from other causes.

- First give the patient a non-narcotic non-steroidal anti-inflammatory drug (NSAID).

- If the patient still feels pain after taking the maximum dose of the NSAID, add a weak opioid narcotic.

- If the patient still feels pain, add a strong opioid narcotic.

At any step, adjuvant analgesics can also be given.

 # Nursing measures for relieving pain

There are several other things you can do to help relieve the patient's pain:

- Talk slowly and quietly with the patient
- Change the position of the patient to make him or her more comfortable
- Place padding over bony areas of the body before you apply a bandage.
- Apply heat or ice to the painful area
- Offer appropriate food
- Give enough fluids

- Encourage visitors to distract and comfort the patient with friendly conversation or by playing favourite music quietly
- Give the patient a warm, relaxing bath
- Give a back rub or massage

> # Believe what the patient tells you about his or her pain.

14

Care of patients in life-threatening emergencies

When the patient's life is in immediate danger, that is an emergency and you need to take urgent action. Emergencies may have many different causes. For example, a person may be badly injured, or suffering a heart attack or stroke, or having a severe allergic reaction. The person may have been poisoned or severely burned, or may be drowning. This chapter focuses on danger signs to look for and immediate measures to take in emergency situations.

Being prepared for emergencies

You should have immediate access to a resuscitation kit or trolley that includes the following:

- syringes, needles (different sizes), butterfly needles (if possible), swabs, strapping (plaster), and an ampoule file (if possible)
- Intravenous (IV) drip sets and intravenous cannulas
- 4-5 litres of IV fluids: Hartmann's or Ringer's lactate, normal saline, 5% dextrose, plasma
- oxygen, if possible
- suction equipment and catheters

- airway tubes and, if possible, a laryngoscope

- tourniquet

- ambu bag (paediatric and adult) and several different sizes of masks

- drugs: The following drugs should be on the trolley or readily available in the emergency room or casualty area of the hospital - 50% dextrose solution, adrenaline, frusemide (Lasix), diazepam (Valium), hydrocortisone/dexamethasone, phenergen, ergometrine, naloxone (Narcan), insulin, lignocaine, snake bite anti-venom (if available), atropine, aminophylline, anti-malarial drugs, aspirin and antibiotics.

The trolley or kit should be checked daily to make sure that all equipment and supplies are ready for use.

The A, B, C and D of resuscitation

In a life-threatening situation, the first task is to resuscitate the patient. Always begin resuscitation at once; do not wait until you have assessed the patient. Follow the A, B, C, and D of resuscitation.

A   Ensure a clear airway

First check to see whether the person's airway is open. If the patient can speak, the airway is clear. If the person cannot speak, see whether the chest wall is expanding. Listen for airway exchange (breathing) and try to feel any breath against your hand. If there is too little or no air movement in a conscious person, the person may be choking.

Airway obstruction: conscious person

If a conscious person is choking, perform the Heimlich manoeuvre. Stand behind the patient, put your arms around the abdomen, between the waist and ribcage, and grasp your hands together. Then give a quick, sudden pull on your hands in an upward thrust. Repeat this squeezing action three or four times if necessary. This will help to dislodge anything caught in the person's airway.

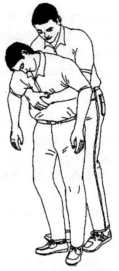

Heimlich manoeuvre

Airway obstruction: unconscious person

If the patient who has choked is unconscious, straddle the patient, (who should be lying on his or her back), and place the heel of your hand in the patient's midline, above the umbilicus and well below the lower sternum. Put your other hand on top of this hand and press inward and upward towards the patient's diaphragm with five quick thrusts. This should dislodge any foreign body in the airway.

If the patient is a child, use the same procedures as for an adult. Repeat the upward thrusts five times.

If the patient is an infant, lay the infant face down on your forearm, with the head lower than the body. Support the infant's head and chest and give five firm slaps between the shoulder blades.

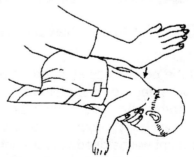

Removing an obstruction from an infant's airway

If this does not dislodge the blockage, place the infant on his or her back with the head lower than the body. Using the first two fingers of one hand, press between the umbilicus and the breast bone with a firm quick movement, five times.

If the patient is not obviously choking, you can probably open the airway by extending the patient's neck. To do so, tilt the head back with one hand and lift the jaw with the other.

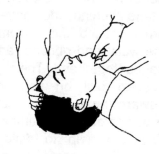

If the patient is unconscious and breathing, put him or her in the coma position, lying on one side with one knee flexed and the head turned sideways. This will prevent either the tongue or vomit from blocking the airway.

Open the airway by tilting head back and lifting chin

Clinical alert: **If it is possible that the spine is broken, do not move the patient at all. Do not extend the neck. Place yourself at the patient's head and open the airway by pushing the angles of the patient's lower jaw forward, while you stabilize the head between your forearms. You may need to use suction to clear the patient's airway.**

B   Ensure that the person is breathing

If the person has stopped breathing, you need to help him or her to breathe after you have cleared the airway. Without breathing, the patient will be dead in four minutes.

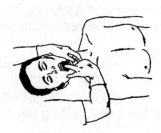

Clearing the airway

Use mouth-to-mouth resuscitation or an ambu bag and mask. Lay the person face up, gently tilt the head back and pull the jaw forward. If the person might have a broken spine, lift the jaw forward at the chin and do not extend the neck.

For mouth-to-mouth resuscitation, pinch the nostrils closed with one hand, open your mouth wide and take a deep breath. Cover the person's mouth with yours and blow strongly into the person's lungs for about two seconds so that the chest rises. Let the air come back out by breaking contact with the patient's mouth, and then blow again. Repeat every five

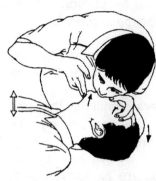

Mouth-to-mouth resuscitation

seconds. For babies or small children, blow gently and repeat every three seconds.

Continue until the person can breathe on his or her own or is clearly dead.

C Ensure that the person's heart is beating

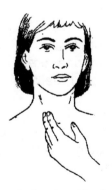

Feeling carotid pulse

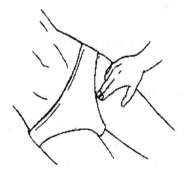

Feeling femoral pulse

If the person is breathing, the heart is beating. If the patient is not breathing, check the carotid pulse (in the neck) or the femoral pulse (inside the upper thigh next to the groin). These are the easiest pulses to feel. In infants, feel for the brachial pulse in the upper, inner arm, between the elbow and shoulder. If there is no pulse and the person is not breathing, begin cardiopulmonary resuscitation (CPR).

The patient should be lying flat on a hard surface. If you suspect spinal injury, keep the head and body in a straight line.

Always ventilate the person first, before doing chest compression.

If you are alone, ventilate the adult patient with two slow, deep breaths lasting about two seconds each, as described above. Then compress the person's chest in the middle of the sternum 15 times. To find the correct

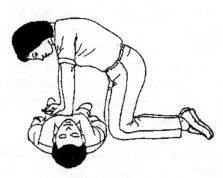

Chest compression

position, first locate the notch or indentation below the sternum, place two fingers above the notch and place your compressing hand above the two fingers. After you have done 15 compressions, ventilate the person with 2 more breaths. Then provide 15 more compressions. Repeat this four times.

If the person is breathing now, monitor closely. If the person is not breathing, continue to ventilate with one breath every 5 to 6 seconds. If there is no pulse or breathing, continue with cardiopulmonary resuscitation.

If there are two people, one can pump the heart 80-100 times a minute while the other ventilates the lungs 12-15 times a minute, or once after every five chest compressions.

196

For cardiopulmonary resuscitation with children, compress the sternum using only one hand at a rate of 80-100 times a minute and ventilate the child once every five compressions.

For infants, use two fingers to compress the chest 100 times a minute and ventilate once every 5 compressions. Compress the chest over the sternum, one finger breadth

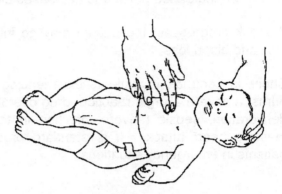

Chest compression of infant

(width) below an imaginary line drawn between the infant's nipples.

If the heart is beating but the patient's pulse is very weak, raise the patient's legs and begin intravenous fluids. Check the blood pressure. Prepare to begin chest compressions if needed.

D   Use a drip to ensure that the person is hydrated and prepare to administer ordered drugs.

The patient may go into shock if there has been too little blood to the vital organs in the body. The signs of shock are:

- anxiety, restlessness or fear

- inability to concentrate

- fast breathing

- thirst, nausea

- dilated pupils

- pale and cool or cold skin

- delayed capillary refilling
- increased pulse and decreased blood pressure.

If shock progresses, the patient may go into a coma or die from fluid and blood loss.

Shock is common in patients experiencing severe injury, severe burns, a severe allergic reaction, drug overdose, poisoning, severe dehydration, sepsis (severe infection in the bloodstream), or a massive heart attack. It is standard practice to give fluids to patients in emergency situations.

 # How to manage shock

- Run an intravenous drip rapidly using normal saline, Hartmann's or plasma; use 5% dextrose solution if nothing else is available.

- Lay the person flat and elevate the legs to help venous blood return to the heart and increase blood pressure. Do not move the patient if spinal cord injury is suspected.

> *Clinical alert:* **Do not raise the legs if the person has congestive heart failure, fluid in the lungs (pulmonary oedema) or severe difficulty breathing (respiratory distress).**

- Continue the intravenous drip until the patient's blood pressure is normal.

Clinical alert: **Do not give fluid to a head injury patient unless he or she is in shock, because the fluid may increase swelling in the brain (cerebral oedema). Be careful not to give too much fluid to cardiac failure patients or children. Some people suggest delaying fluids for persons with trauma.**

- Keep the patient warm.
- Give oxygen if it is available.
- Monitor the patient's airway, breathing and vital signs.

 # How to manage bleeding

If the patient is bleeding, stop the bleeding using a pressure bandage or manual pressure directly over the wound. **Pressure will almost always stop the bleeding.**

Raise the wound above the level of the heart, if possible.

Stop bleeding with pressure dressing

If necessary, apply direct pressure over pressure points such as over the main arteries (brachial in the inner arm or femoral in the upper thigh/groin).

Sometimes a bleeding artery or vein is clearly visible in the wound. If pressure does not stop the bleeding, you can clamp the blood vessel with an artery forceps. Be extremely careful that you do not clamp a vital structure by mistake.

> ***Clinical alert:*** **Tourniquets are dangerous and should not be used to stop bleeding. The only time you ever use a tourniquet is for a wound of the lower limb where the profuse bleeding is life threatening. In this case, release the tourniquet for a few minutes every half hour.**

 # Establish the diagnosis of the patient

Once you have resuscitated the patient and stopped the bleeding, check for the underlying cause of the emergency and begin treatment. Take a brief, focused history and check vital signs.

Head and neck

Check the head for wounds or lacerations, drainage from the nose or ears, mouth and jaw injuries.

Look for swelling or injury to the neck.

Smell the patient's breath for any unusual odour.

Continue to monitor vital signs and assess the patient's level of consciousness. Keep an unconscious patient lying on his or her side.

If there is injury to the eye, cover the eye with a patch.

Check the pupils in both eyes. Normally they are equally round and react when a light is shined in them.

If the nose is bleeding, have the patient sit up if possible and pinch the nose for ten minutes to stop the bleeding.

Shoulders and arms

Check the patient's shoulders, arms and hands. Have the person grip your hands and release, if he or she is able to. Check the range of motion of the elbow. If there are fractures, splint them.

Chest

Check the patient's chest. The chest should expand equally on both sides when the patient breathes.

Look for a sucking chest wound.

Listen to breath sounds from both lungs with the stethoscope, and listen to heart sounds. The lung sounds should be equal on both sides.

Feel the clavicles, sternum and ribs and ask if this causes pain.

If the chest is open, cover the wound with a clean airtight dressing and bandage. If the patient has trouble breathing, untape one edge of the dressing so it acts as a valve.

Abdomen

Assess the abdomen for distension and injury. If you suspect damage to internal organs, or if the abdomen is very tender or rigid, continue intravenous fluids. Do not give anything by mouth because surgery may be necessary.

Spine

If there is a spine injury, do not move the patient until you have at least three people to assist. The patient's neck and spine and trunk must not bend when he or she is moved. While waiting for help, place your hand gently under the lower curve of the back and feel for any tenderness or deformity.

Lower extremities

Examine and feel (palpate) the pelvic area and bones. Look for any obvious injuries.

Examine the legs and feet for deformities, bleeding, bony protrusions, swelling or discolouration.

Check pulses in feet.

 # Emergency treatment

After confirmation of diagnosis, give emergency treatment. If no doctor is available, it may be necessary to arrange for transport of the patient to another health facility.

Immediate drug treatment is essential for certain conditions:

The following drugs should be used according to the treatment schedule (or protocols) established for your health facility.

- For convulsions: Diazepam (Valium)
- For postpartum haemorrhage: Ergometrine
- For asthma: Aminophylline
- For narcotic drug overdose: Narcan

- For patients in severe shock or having an allergic reaction: Intravenous or intramuscular hydrocortisone (plus adrenaline if shock is caused by an allergic reaction)

- For acute allergic reaction: Adrenaline and phenergen

- For pulmonary oedema and cardiac failure: Frusemide (Lasix)

- For insecticide poisoning: Atropine

- For low blood sugar: 50% dextrose solution

- For diabetic hyperglycaemia: Insulin

- For snake bite: Snake bite anti-venom

- For heart attack: Aspirin and thrombolytics, if available. Intravenous morphine may be given for severe pain.

- For infections such as typhoid, meningitis, septicaemia, pelvic inflammatory disease, pneumonia and peritonitis: antibiotics.

- For malaria: Antimalarial drugs such as quinine and chloroquine.

Patients with most of these conditions will need early insertion of an intravenous line

For immediate treatment of a burn, immerse the body part in cold water for the first 30 minutes and give pain medication.

 # Communicate with the family

When the patient is in a life-threatening condition, family members need to be informed as soon as possible. Tell the family what happened, in the order in which the events occurred. Finish by telling the family what the patient's condition is now. If the patient is in a critical condition, it is useful to add something like, "He is not awake and is in no pain." If the patient is dying, try to give the family some advance warning of what to expect.

If the patient is in the emergency room or the operating theatre, or if the family should not come into the patient's room, make them comfortable in a waiting area when they arrive and give them information about the patient as often and as quickly as possible. As soon as possible, allow one family member to see the patient if he or she would like that, but explain what will be seen.

If the patient dies, allow the family to see the patient after death. Before they come in the room, make the body look as natural as possible. Place the body flat, with arms at the sides. Close the eyelids and mouth. Wash soiled areas of the body and cover with a sheet. Remove equipment and supplies from the bedside.

Allow the family to stay as long as they would like to say goodbye to the patient. Provide comfort and care to the family.

15

Care for the dying patient and the family

When it is not possible to prevent a patient dying, and medical care is no longer possible or useful, the nurse provides supportive care to the patient and family. The main goals are to:

- keep the patient comfortable and free of pain
- make the patient's final days as good as possible for both patient and family, with as little suffering as possible
- help the patient to die peacefully
- provide comfort to the family.

It is important for nurses who care for the dying to be aware of their own feelings about death and about their patients. It is difficult to see people die who you have cared for. It is especially difficult if a child or young person dies. You have not only cared for them, you have also cared about them. Many nurses feel frustration and grief when their patients die. It is important for you to recognize those feelings. You need to comfort and support each other in your care of the dying.

Relieve the dying person's pain

Measures to relieve pain are described fully in the chapter on caring for the patient in pain. With patients who are in the last stages of illness, it is essential to remember that one of the main goals of nursing is to relieve or stop suffering. The following guidelines will be helpful.

- Always trust what patients say about their pain. Never just make your own decision about how much pain they are suffering.

- Many patients fear that they will die in agony. Be kind when people express or show fear. Comfort them and tell them that you can take care of the pain and that they do not need to fear.

- Give doses of pain medication that give the most pain control with the least side-effects.

- Give pain medication all through the day and night (around the clock) to make sure that the patient has enough pain relief.

- The best pain medication for the dying is morphine. It can be given in increasing doses as the patient develops tolerance and as its effectiveness is reduced.

> *Clinical alert*: **Do not hesitate to give effective doses of pain medication.**

- Giving some drugs together (in combination) increases their effectiveness. For example, non-steroidal anti-inflammatory drugs increase the effectiveness of opioids like morphine.

- Use the simplest route to give medicine. Give it by mouth, as long as the person can swallow. If the person cannot swallow, repeated boluses of opioids can be given under the skin (the subcutaneous route). Intramuscular routes are not as effective.

- Use other ways to control pain, including massage, music, and comfortable positioning of the patient. Sometimes a hot pad or hot water bottle is helpful with pain.

- Addiction to medication is never important for dying patients.

- Reduced breathing (respiratory depression) is not important for dying patients.

 ## Keep the patient comfortable

- The patient may suffer other discomfort, partly as a result of pain medication.

- If the patient is constipated, a laxative may be helpful. Also encourage the patient to drink fruit juices.

- As much as possible, give the patient a high-calorie, high-vitamin diet. Do not force the patient to eat. The patient should eat only what foods he or she wishes to eat.

- Encourage the patient to drink fluids.

- Keep the patient clean; give frequent baths, give mouth care if the mouth is dry, and clean the eyelids if secretions collect.

- Help the patient to get out of bed and sit in a chair if he or she is able. If not, change the position every two hours and try to keep the patient in whatever positions are most comfortable.

- If the patient has trouble breathing, help him or her to sit up a little.

- If the airway is obstructed, you may need to suction the patient's throat.

- If the patient feels short of breath or gasps for air, give oxygen.

- Even when patients are close to death, they can hear, so do not speak in a whisper. Speak clearly. The patient will also still feel your touch.

How to help the patient to a peaceful death

It is important to ask the patient and family whether the patient would prefer to stay in the hospital or to go home for the last days. Sometimes the family are not able to care for the patient at home, but often there is a choice. If the patient wants to go home, teach the family how to care for him or her. In particular, show the family how to give medication for pain. Make sure that they understand that it is very important to give the medicine in the right dose at the right times. Also explain to them how to make the patient comfortable, as listed above.

If the patient stays in the hospital, try, as much as possible, to do what he or she and the family want. It is important to provide physical comfort. It is also important to make the patient feel secure to calm any fears, and give him or her hope.

Make the person feel safe and secure by showing that he or she will be taken care of, and will not be left alone.

Calm any fears by assuring the patient that he or she will not suffer or die alone.

Give hope. Do not give false reassurances. Give smaller targets. Talk about the future of the patient's family, or suggest that the patient can hope for a good day tomorrow, or remind him or her that the children will soon be visiting.

If the patient has unfinished business, give help with what he or she needs to do. The patient might need help with arrangements for his or her children or house.

Provide spiritual care if the patient wishes, or speak to the family about having the priest or pastor or other religious leader visit.

Above all, respect the patient's decisions. Accept the patient's feelings. If he or she does not want to eat, or get out of bed, or be turned in bed, accept it. Listen and allow the person to talk about how he or she feels. If the patient or family are angry, try to accept it.

Make it easy for the family to stay with the patient as much as they want. Show them how to take care of the patient and keep him or her clean and comfortable.

Keep the family informed about how the patient is. When death is near, let them know so that they can be with the patient at the time of death if they wish.

Care after death

If the family are there at the death, allow them to stay with the patient after death, to say goodbye.

If the family are not there, but would like to see the body after death, make the person look as natural as possible. Make the environment clean. It is important to do this immediately, since the body will start to stiffen (rigor mortis) about two to four hours after death.

Put the body in a flat position on the back, arms at the sides. Put a pillow or rolled towel under the head so that blood does not discolour the face. Close the eyelids and hold them in place for a few seconds so that they will remain closed. Close the mouth. Wash soiled areas of the body. Take away all equipment and supplies from the bedside.

Comfort the family and let them grieve.

16 Preparing the patient for discharge

Start to prepare the patient for return home (discharge) as soon as possible.

The purpose of discharge planning

You need to plan the patient's discharge. The aims are:

- increase the patient's and family's understanding of the health problems and possible complications and restrictions the patient will have at home

- develop the patient's and family's ability to care for the patient's needs and provide a safe environment for the patient at home

- make sure that any referrals needed for further care are properly made.

To begin planning for discharge, look at the problems the patient will have and the care he or she will need. Sometimes people are discharged very quickly from the hospital and still need a lot of care at home. For example, the patient may have a surgical wound that needs to be cared for. Sometimes the patient or family members can take care of everything if they have proper instruction and supplies. At other times the patient will need a nurse to come in and give care at home.

Your preparation of the patient and family will depend on what problems you expect the patient to have at home. Sometimes patients leave the hospital with no problems and no need for further care. In this case, simply make sure that the patient and family understand the possibility of further problems. Tell them what to look for and what to do if there are problems.

In most cases, the patient will need care once he or she leaves the hospital. Talk to the patient as early as possible to find out whether there is someone at home to help. Find out who that person is. Once you know something about the patient's arrangements for care at home, you need to teach the patient and the caregivers what to do at home.

> **Discharge planning should involve both the patient and the family member or other person who will be taking care of the patient.**

 ## Prepare the patient to go home

Ask the patient to have the primary caregiver at home come into the hospital so that you can talk to them together.

Teach the patient and family member about how to handle the care at home. Make sure the patient and family understand what the problems are. Tell them what is likely to happen and when they can expect full recovery. Tell them how to recognize possible problems, and what to do if they see these signs.

Tell the patient and family what the patient can and cannot do. For example, the patient may be on bed rest for three days, or may need to get up every day and walk a few steps. The patient may need to take only a partial bath until bandages are removed. He or she may need to raise a leg or arm for a period of time. The patient may only be able to eat soft food for a few days.

Discuss with the patient and family what they may need to do to make the home safer and easier for the patient. If the patient sleeps far from the bathroom or latrine and is not yet able to walk well, the patient may need to keep a container at the bedside until he or she can walk easily. If the patient will be unsteady, he or she may need a cane.

Tell the patient and family about the medications the patient will need to take. Make sure that they understand when to take them and how much to take. Make sure that the patient and family understand how long to take the medications. Sometimes patients stop taking their medicines when they feel better if they do not understand that they must continue them. Sometimes patients do not know that they will need to have a prescription for more supplies of medicine. Explain to the patient and family if the medicines need to be taken with food, or need to be taken an hour before meals.

Discuss the need for adequate fluids and a nutritious diet. If the patient is still on fluids only, tell the family when and how to move onto soft foods and a normal diet. Tell the patient and family that the signs of drinking enough fluids are moist (not dry) lips and tongue, regular urination and urine that is clear, not cloudy.

It is particularly important to give the patient and family clear instructions for dealing with the patient's pain. Try to help the patient to work out a medication schedule that will not require getting up in the night. Pain is less if medications are given regularly, on schedule. Make sure that the patient understands that he or she should continue using the medicine until the pain has really stopped. Explain that pain is controlled better if medications are taken before pain becomes severe.

Give the patient the materials or equipment he or she will need or give instructions about how to get what is needed. Tell the patient clearly what to do. Give instructions in writing as well, as it is easy to forget details, especially if the patient is upset. Teach the patient or family member how to do any needed procedures. Check that they understand by asking them to show you how to do the procedure. This is called a return demonstration.

If the patient will be on bed rest, teach the family how to position the patient in bed, turn him or her, and help the patient move from the bed to a chair. Family members often do not know how vitally important it is to turn the patient regularly, to help him or her to get out of bed and into a chair, and then help with walking if the patient is ready. Tell the family that proper positioning and turning will make the patient much more comfortable and will prevent bedsores. Also, if the family understand how to move the patient without harming him or her, they will be more confident in giving care.

> **Family caregivers can learn to give care by helping you with the activities, then doing them while you watch.**

Talk carefully to the patient and family about home remedies and traditional healers. It is important to know whether the patient is being treated by a traditional healer or being given home remedies. Do not criticize the family for using traditional healing methods if these are not harmful to the patient. Many traditional healing methods are effective. For example, if the patient catches a cold, herbal teas work as well as strong medicines or cough syrups. Encourage the family to tell you or the doctor if the patient has a serious health problem.

If the patient needs follow-up care at home, make the referral before the patient leaves the hospital. In small communities the nurse who cared for the patient in hospital may be the nurse who gives home care. But it is usually a community health nurse who provides home care. It is important for the hospital nurse to refer patients to the community health nurse soon after the patient comes into hospital. It is very helpful if the community health nurse can meet the patient and family before the patient is discharged. Tell the patient how to contact the nurse in case the nurse does not come or if there is any confusion about time and place.

Find out about the social services available in the community and refer the patient when necessary.

Basic principles of good patient teaching

When preparing the patient and family for discharge, always follow the basic principles of good patient teaching:

- Schedule the teaching when the patient will be alert and interested in learning.

- Start with the thing that the patient is most concerned about.

- If you have a number of things to tell the patient, always begin with the simplest information. Next give the patient the more complicated information.

- Use clear, ordinary words, not medical words.

- Stop if the patient looks puzzled and ask if he or she understands.

- If necessary, say the information again, or say it in different words until you are sure that he or she understands you.

- Encourage the patient to comment and ask questions, and to show you what he or she knows.

- Ask for return demonstrations of procedures the patient will need to carry out. If procedures involve personal areas of the body, it may be helpful to ask a nurse of the same sex as the patient to show him or her how to do them.

- Encourage the family members to ask questions. Make sure that they understand what will need to be done.

- Use pictures in your teaching and give simple handouts in the patient's language.

- Give clear answers to questions and give as much comfort and reassurance as possible, without saying something which is not true.

 # When the patient leaves the hospital

- When the patient is leaving the hospital, again go over the information you have given earlier and the doctor's orders for medications, treatments, or special equipment.

- Go over the referral appointments so that the patient is clear about what to do.

- Make sure the patient and family understand the patient's limitations, how long these will go on, how to recognize warning signs and symptoms, and the actions they should take to help the patient's recovery as much as possible.

- Encourage the patient and family to come back to the hospital if his or her condition is not improving or is getting worse.

- When the patient has recovered, encourage a return to normal life and responsibilities.

REFERENCES

WHO Publications

Action Programme for the Elimination of Leprosy: Status Report 1996. Geneva: World Health Organization, 1996 (WHO/LEP/96.5).

AIDS Home Care Handbook. Geneva: World Health Organization, 1993 (WHO/GPA/IDS/HCS/93.2).

Chemotherapy of Leprosy. Report of a WHO Study Group. Geneva: WHO Technical Report Series 847, 1994.

Caring for Mothers and Their Babies. Manila, Philippines: World Health Organization Regional Office for the Western Pacific, 1997.

Clean Delivery: Techniques and Practices for Prevention of Tetanus and Sepsis. Geneva: World Health Organization, 1994 (WHO/MSM/CHD94.6).

Community Health Worker: Working Guide, Guidelines for Training, Guidelines for Adaptation. Geneva: World Health Organization, 1990.

Counselling for Maternal and Child Health. Manila, Philippines: WHO Regional Office for the Western Pacific, 1995.

Detecting Pre-Eclampsia: Using and Maintaining Blood Pressure Equipment. Geneva: World Health Organization, 1992 (WHO/MCH/MSM/92.3).

Diarrhoea Management Training Course: Participant Manual. (Rev. Ed.). Geneva: World Health Organization, 1992 (CDD/SER/90.2. Rev 1).

Elimination of Leprosy (Revised ed.). Geneva: World Health Organization, 1996 (WHO/LEP/96.4).

Epidemiological Review of Leprosy in the Western Pacific Region 1982-1995. Manila, Philippines: WHO Regional Office for the Western Pacific, 1996.

Epidemiological Review of Tuberculosis in the Western Pacific Region. Manila, Philippines: Research Institute of Tuberculosis, Japan Anti-Tuberculosis Association and WHO Regional Office for the Western Pacific, 1995.

Essential Elements of Obstetric Care at First Referral Level. Geneva: World Health Organization, 1991.

Guide to Eliminating Leprosy as a Public Health Problem. (Pocket Ed.). Geneva: World Health Organization, 1995 (WHO/LEP/95.1).

Guidelines for Cholera Control. Geneva: World Health Organization, 1993.

Guidelines for the Clinical Management of HIV Infection in Adults. Geneva: World Health Organization, 1991 (WHO/GPA/IDS/HCS/91.6).

Harries, A.D., & Maher, D. *TB/HIV: A Clinical Manual.* Geneva: World Health Organization, 1996.

HIV Infection and AIDS: Guidelines for Nursing Care. HIV/AIDS Reference Library for Nurses, Vol. 4. Manila, Philippines: WHO Regional Office for the Western Pacific, 1993.

HIV Prevention and Care: Teaching Modules for Nurses and Midwives. Geneva: World Health Organization, 1993 (WHO/GPA/CNP/TMD/93.3).

Infection Control. HIV/AIDS Reference Library for Nurses, Vol. 2. Manila, Philippines: WHO Regional Office for the Western Pacific, 1993.

Intercountry Workshop on the Role of Nurses and Auxiliary Staff in Care of Persons with HIV/AIDS/STD. Alexandria, Egypt: WHO Regional Office for the Eastern Mediterranean, 1997.

Learning Material on Nursing (LEMON), Chapters 1-13. Copenhagen, Denmark: WHO Regional Office for Europe, 1996.

Living with AIDS in the Community. Geneva: World Health Organization, 1992 (WHO/GPA/IDS/HSC/92.1).

Management and Prevention of Diarrhoea: Practical Guidelines (3rd Ed.). Geneva: World Health Organization, 1993.

Management of Acute Respiratory Infections in Children. Geneva: World Health Organization, 1995.

Managing Maternal and Child Health Programmes: A Practical Guide. Manila: WHO Regional Office for the Western Pacific, 1997.

MDT: Questions and Answers (Revised edition). Geneva: World Health Organization, 1996 (WHO/LEP/96.6).

Mother-Baby Package: Implementing Safe Motherhood in Countries. Geneva: World Health Organization, 1994 (WHO/FHE/MSM/94.11).

Obstetric and Contraceptive Surgery at the District Hospital: A Practical Guide. Geneva: World Health Organization, WHO/MCH/MSM/92.8.

On Being in Charge: A Guide to Management in Primary Health Care. (2nd Ed.). Geneva: World Health Organization, 1992.

Outpatient Management of Young Children with ARI: A Four-Day Clinical Course: Director's and Facilitator's Guide. Geneva: World Health Organization, 1995.

Outpatient Management of Young Children with ARI: A Four-Day Clinical Course. Participant Manual. Geneva: World Health Organization, 1995.

Quality Health Care for the Elderly: A Manual for Instructors of Nurses and Other Health Workers. Manila: WHO Regional Office for the Western Pacific, 1995.

TB: WHO Report on the Tuberculosis Epidemic. Geneva: World Health Organization, 1997.

Things to Do to Stay Healthy. Manila: WHO Regional Office for the Western Pacific, 1995.

Other Publications

Balladin, B., Hart, R., Huenges, R., & Versluys, Z., *Child Health. Rural Health Series 1.* Nairobi, Kenya: African Medical and Research Foundation, 1984.

Cage, C.B., Francis, M.D., Van Leuven, K., & White, C.T., *Clinical Companion to Fundamentals of Nursing Care.* Redwood City, CA, USA: Addison-Wesley, 1995.

Child Health Dialogue, 2nd and 3rd quarters, double issue 3 and 4, 1996.

Child Health Dialogue, 4th quarter, Issue 5, 1996.

Chin, P., *Fundamentals of Nursing.* El Paso, Texas, USA: Skidmore-Roth Publishing, Inc, 1995.

Crofton, J., Horne, N., & Miller, F., *Clinical Tuberculosis.* London, England: Macmillan Education, Ltd., 1992.

Desenclos, J.C. (Ed.), *Clinical Guidelines: Diagnostic and Treatment Manual* (3rd Ed.). Paris, France: Medicins sans Frontieres, 1993.

Ebrahim, G. J., *Nutrition in Mother and Child Health.* London, England: Macmillan, 1983.

Ebrahim, G. J., *Paediatric Practice in Developing Countries.* (2nd Ed.). London, England: Macmillan, 1993.

Essential Obstetrics Function. Kathmandu, Nepal: Health Learning Materials Centre, T.U. Institute of Medicine, 1993.

Evian, C., Orlek, J., & Scholtz, A., *Primary Clinical Care, Books 1-14.* Johannesburg, South Africa: Health Services Development Unit, Department of Community Health, University of the Witwatersrand Medical School, 1987-1992.

Eye Infections. *The Prescriber: Guidelines on the Rational Use of Drugs in Basic Health Services,* Issue no. 13. New York, NY, USA: UNICEF, 1997.

Hosken, F., *The Universal Childbirth Picture Book.* Lexington, MA, USA: Women's International Network News, 1995.

Infection Prevention Policy Guidelines for Health Facilities. Port Moresby, Papua New Guinea: National Department of Health, 1995.

Kenyon, M., *Maternal Child Health Manual for Solomon Islands.* Honiara, Solomon Islands: Save the Children Fund Australia, 1992.

King, M., King, F., & Soebagio, M., *Primary Child Care: A Manual for Health Workers , Book One.* Oxford, England: Oxford University Press, 1984.

Klein, S., *A Book for Midwives.* Palo Alto, CA, USA: The Hesperian Foundation, 1995.

Kozier, B., Erb, G., Blais, K, & Wilkinson, J., *Fundamentals of Nursing Care: Concepts, Process, and Practice* (5th Ed.). Redwood City, CA, USA: Addison Wesley, 1995.

Luckman, J. (Ed.), *Saunders Manual of Nursing Care.* Philadelphia, PA: Saunders, 1997.

Midwives Manual on Maternal Care. San Lazaro, Manila: Maternal and Child Health Service, Department of Health, and UNICEF, 1993.

Practical Guidelines for Preventing Infections Transmitted by Blood or Air in Health-Care Settings. London: Appropriate Health Resources and Technologies Action Group, 1996.

Ramanujam, T.M., *Parenteral Nutrition in Infants and Children.* Madras, India: V.V. Publishers, 1988.

Reducing the Impact of HIV/AIDS on Nursing/Midwifery Personnel: Guidelines for National Nurses' Associations and Others. Geneva: International Council of Nurses, 1996.

Rigal, J. Ed., *Minor Surgical Procedures in Remote Areas.* Paris: Medecins sans Frontieres, 1989.

Werner, D., & Bower, B., *Helping Health Workers Learn.* Palo Alto, CA: The Hesperian Foundation, 1982.

Werner, D., Thurman, C., & Maxwell, J., *Where There Is No Doctor.* (Revised Ed.). Palo Alto, CA: The Hesperian Foundation, 1992.

Witter Du Gas, B., *Introduction to Patient Care.* (4th Ed.). Philadelphia: Saunders, 1983.